HARVARD UNIVERSITY EXTENSION SCHOOL

SSCI S-100A
Proseminar: Graduate Research Methods and Scholarly Writing in the Social Sciences
Psychology and Anthropology
Literature Review

Merging Childcare and Senior-care to Provide the Healthier Psychological Environment for Healthcare Treatments.

Kim Byrd-Rider

7/10/18

TABLE OF CONTENTS

Introduction

The children of America are America's future but, arguably, the geriatrics of America are America's future too. America has given up on the societal contribution ability of the geriatric community. Geriatric people are gathered together and encouraged to go into nursing homes or senior living facilities/neighborhoods. Some live secluded and alone. Whole communities, the size of cities, are now dedicated to senior living. Shopping malls, hospitals and golf courses thrive within them for the geriatrics' pleasure. Step down programs are available when the geriatric person's health deteriorates, enabling the person to stay in the familiar community. Aligned with the movie "Stepford Wives", these communities revolve around familiarity, stability and pleasure: the ultimate American retirement goal. As outlined here, it is the really the ultimate trap into hedonism.

Background

Physical therapy is provided in a clinical setting. Seniors are lonely and board and bond with the therapist. PTs have to release them. Seniors still not developing relationship bonds. We keep children and seniors separate

The Problem

To quote renowned anthropologist Jason Throop (2010), "To be human is to be vulnerable to both the possibility and inevitability of suffering pain. Woven into the fabric of our existence, pain is an experience that calls forth questions of meaning, morality, despair, and hope."

The psychological component of pain and PTs' inability to do that.

The over 60 years old crowd is exploding worldwide. By 2050, the number will rise from 605 million in 2015 to 2 billion (Offord, Wyrko, Downes, Hopper, Harriman, & Gordon, 2016). People over 80 years is expected to quadruple up to 395 million in that timeframe. In the United Kingdom (UK) the senior population accounts for two-thirds of acute care hospital admissions. (Offord, et al., 2016). For general practice the highest consultation rate is for people 85-89 years old. Elective surgeries like knee replacements is rising. The World Health Organization is making this problem their global healthcare priority and is discussing policy, health services structures, frontline care delivery and workforce reconfiguration (Offord, et al., 2016).

Even if hospitals could retain all of their current employees, they are predicted to become extremely short of employees due to growing elderly populations and increasing healthcare complexity (Canadian Nurses Association, 2009). Starting 2022, the Canadian Nurses Association (2009) predicts that, like most other countries, they will be short 60,000 nurses. In 2015, hospitals averaged an ongoing 7% nursing vacancy rate (University of New Mexico, 2016). The PT jobs are expected to grow by 28% between 2016 and 2026 due to the growth in aging baby-boomer numbers, elective joint surgeries, strokes, diabetes and obesity (Bureau of Labor and Statistics, 2018). This is a larger amount than any other occupation (Bureau of Labor and Statistics, 2018).

We have to find a better way to improve senior health to take the stressors off of the healthcare system. Soon seniors will be waiting on lists for months to get a doctor's appointment, if this is not already occurring.

Hypotheses

Seniors will improve faster and more from pain symptoms when PTs treat them in an intergenerational environment as opposed to being treated in a clinical environment. Pain outcome measurements for seniors will improve more and faster when PTs use mindful treatments and play-oriented functional movement as opposed to traditional physical therapy exercises and functional movement. PTs will be more satisfied with their jobs and less likely to quit their jobs after working in an intergenerational care and mindful treatment, play-oriented environment. Well-being scores will rise in the seniors and PTs post-experiment. Interviews with the children, seniors and PTs at the end of the experiment will show enthusiastic and positive support for the program from all three groups compared to the control group.

Research Question(s)

How and to what extent does an intergenerational environment and mindfulness interventions with play-oriented functional activities improve physical therapy outcomes in geriatric patients?

Literature Review

Literature Genres

Research was gathered using Harvard's Hollis database and Google Scholar database for peer reviewed journal articles and literature reviews. All efforts were made to use journal articles less than four years old but due to some of the topics older research had to be used..

To respond to the research question, this review is divided into topics. The first topic reviews the literature about the current physical therapy conditions and the possible need for change. The three following topics discuss the pros and cons of the elements within the research question: mindful physical therapy interventions, play-oriented functional activity interventions and intergenerational care.

Hundreds of pro-mindfulness articles, two con-mindfulness articles and one healthcare application of a mindfulness program were found. The mindful interventions section is quite long due to the amount and different types of research available. This section is divided into subtopics, accordingly. Contrarily other topics were lacking in research, like seniors' physical health benefits from intergenerational care and play. These sections are much shorter as a result. Knowing the current situation of physical therapy treatments for seniors, those over 55 years of age, will lay the foundation for the needed results of the research question.

Current Physical Therapy Conditions

Definition of terms.

Physical therapists (PTs) work in private offices, clinics, hospitals, patients' homes, schools and nursing homes (Bureau of Labor and Statistics, 2018). According to the American Physical Therapy Association (APTA), the goal of a PT is to "promote the ability to move, reduce pain, restore function and prevent disability (2018, p.1)." They do this by using their graduate-level degreed skill-set to develop fitness and wellness programs for their patients of all ages. The vision statement for the APTA is "Transforming society by optimizing movement to improve the human experience (American Physical Therapy Association, 2018, p.1)." The following is the scope of practice for a PT as outlined by the APTA:

> PTs provide care to patients/ clients of all ages who have impairments, activity limitations, and participation restrictions due to musculoskeletal, neuromuscular, cardiovascular/pulmonary, and/or integumentary disorders. PTs design individualized plans of care based on their clinical judgment and patient/client goals. PTs collaborate with other health care professionals to address patient needs, increase communication, and provide efficient and effective care across the continuum of health care settings. (American Physical Therapy Association, 2011, p.9).

To summarize, a PT's duties are to provide patient care including education for musculoskeletal, neuromuscular, cardiovascular/pulmonary and integumentary disorders. Psychological disorders like anxiety, depression, fear, loneliness and boredom, which accompany many people in pain, are to be referred to a psychologist or counselor, because those diagnoses are within a psychologist's scope of practice.

In the passage above, the APTA says PTs are to "collaborate with other healthcare professionals" for additional healthcare needs. PTs cannot write prescriptions of any sort. If the PT believes a patient needs additional psychological care for pain, they must refer the patient back to the physician who in-turn can refer the patient to a mental health provider. The PT cannot legally recommend mental health directly to the patient. They can only recommend it directly to the doctor for his/her analysis, due to a PTs' practice limitations and inadequate mental health diagnostic skill-set.

Psychological program allowances.

PTs have been trained in the past to deliver a psychological program called Pain Coping Skills Training (PCST) to patients, though (Nielsen, Keefe, Bennell, & Jull, 2014). The PTs' program trainers and mentors were psychologists and the program was shown to be effective for the eight PTs in the study (Nielsen, Keefe, Bennell, & Jull, 2014). After the study, most of the therapist complained that their work environment was not conducive to PCST patient implementation, the PCST treatment was time consuming, and insurance companies would not pay the PTs for psychological treatments because it was not in their scope of practice (Centers for Medicare & Medicaid Services, 2018; Nielsen, Keefe, Bennell, & Jull, 2014). Another barrier in this study was public expectation. Patients did not expect, nor did they feel comfortable, receiving psychological treatments from their PT (Nielsen, Keefe, Bennell, & Jull, 2014). These barriers confound the need for PTs to address the psychological component of pain even the research says it is best-practice (Nielsen, Keefe, Bennell, & Jull, 2014).

Bio-psycho-social model need.

"There is increasing recognition of the benefits of incorporating the bio-psycho-social model of health within physical therapy practices. This increasing recognition reflects a growing understanding of the limitations of purely biomedical approaches in the treatment of chronic musculoskeletal conditions, particularly with regard to pain management (Nielsen, Keefe, Bennell, & Jull, 2014, p.198;) Most of the past research papers agree on this topic. Much of it took place from the 1990s until around 2011, when it was exhausted (Nielsen, Keefe, Bennell, & Jull, 2014). Recent research on the topic is mostly literature reviews of the plethora of earlier literature, like Nielsen and colleagues' paper (2014).

For another example, a 2007 meta-analysis of 27 articles, out of 233 randomized controlled trials found, analyzed psycho-social interventions in arthritis pain management (Dixon, Keefe, Scipio, Perri, & Abernethy, 2007). The measurements observed were pain intensity outcomes, psychological, physical and biological function. Patients receiving psycho-social interventions had significantly lower pain than the controls did. The psycho-social intervention patients also performed better psychologically, physically and functionally than the control group. Of the studies used, 23-24 had high internal and external quality. The mean age was 58.9 years, 69.5% were female and 81% were Caucasian. Traditional cognitive behavior treatments (CBT) for pain management/pain coping skills was the most frequently tested intervention (70%), followed by stress management (15%), psychodynamic intervention (6%), biofeedback (3%), emotional disclosure (3%), and hypnosis (3%). Five studies (15%) tested more than one. The results were varied but patterns in the literature existed. Coping skills improved the most with a large effect size, while anxiety and joint swelling had a medium effect size. A small effect size was found for improvements in depression, psychological disability, pain self-efficacy and physical disability. No significant improvements were found for fatigue and stiffness. The researchers concluded that psychologists should include physical interventions and PTs should include psychological treatments (Dixon, et al., 2007). The problem with this recommendation is that it is not paid for by insurance companies, including Medicare.

Many if not most of the private insurance companies directly replicate the Medicare reimbursement amounts for treatments (George Mason University, 2015). Indirectly, Medicare sets the standards for other insurance companies (George Mason University, 2015). Insurance companies only pay psychologists for psychological interventions and PTs for physical related interventions (Centers for Medicare & Medicaid Services, 2018; Nielsen, Keefe, Bennell, & Jull, 2014). All different types of treatments have an assigned code and the codes billed for must match the provider who billing or payment is rejected (George Mason University, 2015). Not only do PTs have legal issues with giving optimal recommended care, they have personal hurtles that block optimal patient care, too.

Ageism, cynicism and job turnover.

Healthcare professionals experience seniors through a complaining-oriented, disease focused lens which causes negative attitudes towards and stereotypes of geriatric populations (Rubin, 2016). Healthcare professionals develop ageism as a result of listening to the ongoing poor health situations of seniors that come to them for help. An ageism attitude reduces effective care delivery and impacts an older adult's long-term health outcomes (Reyna, Goodwin, & Ferrari, 2007). It also causes healthcare workers to depersonalize from their patients (Anderson, Gould-Fogerite, Pratt, & Perlman, 2015). Healthcare workers' ageism is contributed to a lack of quality time spent with seniors and a personal fear of death and aging (Bodner, 2009). This is a problem because seniors currently comprise the largest population served across all healthcare professions (Wong, Odom, & Barr, 2014).

Depersonalized attitudes towards patients creates burnout and high job turnover for not only PTs but healthcare workers in general. A sample study showed a high turnover rate for PTs. Of 882 nationwide PTs in a one year study, 16% quit their jobs, 2% left the profession and 7% rotated to another position in the company, totaling 25% (Campo, Weiser, & Koenig, 2009). PT turnover rates in nursing homes can be much higher at 85% per year (Physical therapy workforce project, 2008). Comparatively, the national job turnover average according to the U.S. department of Labor is 2.4% (Job openings and labor turnover, 2018). The U.S. department of labor also verified that healthcare job turnover rose during 2018 (Job openings and labor turnover, 2018). In the nationwide PT study, job strain was most associated with job turnover than job demands or job control alone (Physical therapy workforce project, 2008). According to the researchers, job strain was a combination of high demands with low control. Ironically, this study related job strain and job control as a significant indicator for a PT to personally experience work-related musculoskeletal pain but job demands had no pain effects (Physical therapy workforce project, 2008). This is another example of the psychological component of pain and the problem obviously does not only lie with patient's pain.

The American Medical Association and 10 leading healthcare CEO's declared healthcare burnout a public health crisis as of 2017 (Noseworthy, 2017). The Maslach Burnout Inventory (MBI) is a gold standard job-burnout assessment tool used for these types of findings. In a study using the MBI scale and 1,366 PTs (69% female, 92% white; proportional to APTA's membership base), 29% of PTs had high emotional exhaustion and13% had all three burnout symptoms of emotional exhaustion, depersonalization (indifference towards patients), and decreased personal accomplishment (Anderson, Gould-Fogerite, Pratt, & Perlman, 2015).

The authors of the tool, Christina Maslach and colleague (2016) define these constructs in detail. Overwhelming exhaustion is having feelings of wearing out, loss of energy, depletion, debilitation and fatigue. Feelings of cynicism and detachment (depersonalization) from the job evolves negative or inappropriate attitudes towards clients, irritability, loss of idealism and withdrawal. Lastly, ineffective or lack of accomplishment produces feelings of reduced productivity, low morale and inability to cope.

To make the feelings of ineffectiveness and lack of accomplishment worse, PTs have productivity quotas that are continually becoming more demanding and unachievable. A quote from the APTA's industry magazine says, "some facilities have become 'productivity systems,' that attempt to push PTs toward unethical practice to meet their unsubstantiated (high productivity) benchmarks," (Hayhurst, 2015, p. 1).

Cynicism, originally called depersonalization by Maslach and Leiter (2016), negatively effects worker time efficiency, productivity, effort and performance (Kim, et al., 2009). Cynicism increases counterproductive work behaviors (Luksyte, Spitzmeuller, & Maynard,

2011). Cynicism causes employees to cut themselves off from organizational values and other employees which decreases teamwork and cooperation, compromising patient care (Mantler, Godin, Cameron, & Horsburgh, 2015). Once a high level of employee cynicism develops in an organization, it can stay high because it is an attitude. It can also be lowered through organizational effort, according to Boersma and Lindblom (2009) along with Wanous, Reichers and Austin (2000).

These personal healthcare worker deficits build into administration problems, facility financial sustainability problems and profit margin collapses. Turnover costs can add up to millions of dollars per year for large healthcare companies (University of New Mexico, 2016). Even if clinics could retain all of their current employees, they are predicted to become extremely short of employees due to growing elderly populations and increasing healthcare complexity (Canadian Nurses Association, 2009). Physical therapy needs are expect to grow by 28% between 2016 and 2026, more than any other profession in America (Bureau of Labor and Statistics, 2018). Keeping current workers satisfied and employed is paramount for employers to generate income and save job turnover money leakage, not to mention optimal patient quality-care. Mindful programs for the healthcare professionals has shown to decrease job cynicism, job burnout and job turnover (Dane, & Brummel, 2014), increasing a clinic's administrative motivation to place PTs in a more psychologically supportive environment, like an intergenerational care unit using mindful interventions.

Mindful solutions for healthcare workers.

Compassion in patient care is significantly decreasing for healthcare workers. (American Medical Association, *2001*; Institute of Medicine, *2004*; Francis, *2013*; MacLean, *2014*; Willis, 2015). Self-compassion meditations for the healthcare workers and care givers: findings suggest that an 8-week yoga and compassion meditation program can improve the quality of life, vitality, attention, and self-compassion of caregivers (Calder, 2017). Education for self-compassion, emotional intelligence, and mindfulness training need to be incorporated into medical students' curricula and programs to promote healthcare worker and patient well-being (Patsiopoulos & Buchanan, *2011*; Senyuva et al., *2014*; Olson et al., *2015*; Kemper et al., *2015*; Beaumont et al., 2016).

General job-performance research using mindful awareness and concentration interventions are abundant (Glomb, Duffy, Bono & Yang, 2011; Good, Lyddy, Glomb, Bono, Brown, Duffy, ... & Lazar, 2016). Two systematic reviews of the literature generalize the workplace improvement outcomes from mindful programs into three categories: (a) improved worker physical and psychological well-being, (b) improved relationship qualities and (c) improved job performance (Glomb, et al., 2011; Good,et al., 2016). A plethora of research studies support increased work-engagement after mindful awareness and concentration interventions (e.g., Brown, Ryan, & Creswell, 2007; Dane, & Brummel, 2014; Hülsheger, Alberts, Feinholdt, & Lang, 2013; Leroy, Anseel, Dimitrova, & Sels, 2013).

A 10-day daily survey study of a control group of 50 healthcare workers and an experimental healthcare group of 50 people using a self-taught (booklet) on meditation awareness and concentration. Participants were from hospitals, healthcare schools and medical practices in German cities. The researchers found positive outcomes for increased job-satisfaction and less emotional exhaustion (one of the three constructs of job burnout which was found to be high in PTs) among healthcare workers (Hülsheger, Alberts, Feinholdt, & Lang, 2013). If PTs show patients how to do mindful interventions, then they are doing the interventions themselves throughout their entire workday. This means PTs most probably reap the mindful practice benefits while administering mindful interventions to patients.

Mindful Patient Interventions

Definition of terms.

The popularity of mindful techniques has quickly escalated over the last two decades with the support of American physicians like Dr. John Kabat-Zinn. He has provided one of many definitions for mindfulness (2013, 1:02), "Mindfulness is the awareness that arises through paying attention, on purpose, in a very thoughtful way, in the present moment, non-judgmentally and as if your life depends on it." Dr. Kabat-Zinn points out that focusing is the key and it does not matter what is focused on. Not to be confused with relaxing, mindfulness is the training of awareness monitoring (Kabat-Zinn, 2013). Mindful awareness and mindful concentration is also defined as the essence and experience of engagement, the noticing of new things and is what enlivens us (Langer, 2012).

Types of mindfulness include concentration and awareness. Mindful concentration is the fixating on an object (transcendental meditation) like a mantra, breathing, a physical experience or a picture to disengage from thoughts or emotions (Hülsheger, Alberts, Feinholdt, & Lang,

2013). The purpose of mindfulness is to generate deep comfort and focus. Mindful awareness is fixating on the present moment, staying alert and being less judgmental during that moment. One strives to apply acceptance and compassion to observed thoughts and feelings. The aim of successful mindfulness is to break the chain of thought association and to stop reacting to those thoughts (Hülsheger, Alberts, Feinholdt, & Lang, 2013). Mindful concentration and mindful awareness are similar. The mindful practitioner probably alternates between the two no matter which one is intended. Mindful interventions also include exercises like yoga, tai chi, Pilates and Feldenkrais.

Billability.

These mindful exercises fall under the scope of practice for PTs and are paid by Medicare, Medicaid and all other insurances due to their strengthening, stretching and balance components (Centers for Medicare & Medicaid Services, 2018). The Medicare medical codes for the mindful exercises are therapeutic activities, neurological re-education and/or therapeutic exercise depending on the therapist's patient goals for the mindful exercise. Yogic breathing techniques are also billable by PTs due to their skeletal muscle strengthening and stretching of the diaphragm and intercostal muscles plus the dozens of secondary breathing muscles.

Meditation is a mindful practice which is unattended by the therapist. The therapist can be working with another patient while the first person is in meditation. Patients can also perform meditation during unattended electrical stimulation, heat or ice which is chargeable to insurance companies (Centers for Medicare & Medicaid Services, 2018). If a psychologist had patient goals for focus, concentration or breath regulation, they too can charge insurance companies for the same mindful exercises (Centers for Medicare & Medicaid Services, 2018). There is plenty of evidence about the psychological effects, brain effects and physical health effects of mindful programs, as follows.

Psychological health effects.

Self-compassion meditations are showing promise for psychological health effects in the literature. According to psychology professor Dr. Kristin Neff, self-compassion is "extending compassion to one's self in instances of perceived inadequacy, failure, or general suffering. Three main components: (a) self-kindness- being kind and understanding towards oneself in instances of pain or failure rather than being harshly self-critical, (b) common humanity- perceiving one's experiences as part of the larger human experience rather than seeing them as a separating and isolating and (c) mindfulness- holding painful thoughts and feelings in balanced awareness rather than over-identifying with them" (Neff, 2003). Self-compassion meditations increases: self-esteem, successful aging, general well-being, life satisfaction, functioning, resilience and emotion regulation and they also decrease depression, fear of failure, anxiousness, fear of rejection, negative affect, self-pity, catastrophizing, resignation, emotional problems and PTSD symptom severity(Allen & Leary, 2010; Leary, Tate, Adams, Allen, & Hancock, 2007; Neff, 2003; Neff, Kirkpatrick, & Rude, 2007; Scolglio, 2015).

Patients often ignore doctors' recommendations, fume about the inconvenience of being incapacitated, and blame themselves for the illness or injury (Putnam, Finney, Barkley, & Bonner, 1994). People's attention is derailed by judgmental, defensive, or otherwise non-self-compassionate thoughts (Greeson & Brantley, 2009; Shapiro & Schwartz, 1999) The psychologically calming properties of the vagus nerve is the core component of the parasympathetic nervous system (PNS) and is the central player of Porges's Polyvagal Theory (2007). The theory demonstrates positive correlations between (a) positive emotions and affect, (b) high vagal tone and (c) perceived positive social connections. Each influences the other in an upward positive spiral improving psychological and even physical health (Kok & Fredrickson, 2010).

What does the vagus nerve have to do with social interactions? The vagus nerve links to nerves coordinating eye gaze, facial expressions and tuning into human voices (Porges, 2007). Vagus nerve tone reciprocally increases form intranasal oxytocin produced by positive social engagement (Kemp et al., 2012). So, high vagal tone is associated with prosocial behavior (Fabes, Eisenberg, & Eisenbud, 1993) and social closeness (Kok & Fredrickson, 2010). High vagal nerve tone can be measured quantifiably. The 10th cranial nerve (the vagus nerve) registers low tone when the "fight or flight" sympathetic nervous system (SNS) operates and high tone when the "rest and relax" PNS operates. Together the SNS and PNS are the autonomic nervous system, which is responsible for unconscious bodily functions like breathing, heart rate and digestion. The practical question is: What interventions kick start the positive movement of any of the three of Porges's Polyvagal Theory (2007) to encourage the positive upward spiral of all three: positive emotions and affect, high vagal tone and perceived positive social connections.

According to a lecture produced by the Harvard Medical School, there are four categories of mindful interventions (2008). Two of them fall into the sub-category of *concentration type mindfulness*: (a) concentrating with focused attention on an image, a sound (mantra) or a single-pointed object (body part, breath); (b) ethical enhancement like practicing loving kindness, compassion or forgiveness. The other two are in the sub-category of *awareness type mindfulness*: (c) receptive work or open monitoring awareness like diffusing attention toward any object that arises naturally or mental noting/labeling; and (d) *awareness monitoring or mindful movements* like yoga, tai chi and qi gong (Harvard Medical School, 2008). Let's examine the positive and adverse effects of mindful interventions in the research.

Positive effects.

Mindful activities contribute to five areas of significantly measurable improvement in the well-being of the mind, according to a Harvard Medical School lecture (2008, lecture): (a) intention (motivation makes a difference); (b) attention regulation (stability, control, and clarity); (c) emotion regulation (response inhibition and equanimity); (d) extinction and reconsolidation (of sensory-affective-motor scripts/schemas/biases); and (e) pro-sociality (empathy, ethical framework in social cognition).

Mindfulness positively correlates to increases in happiness, relationship satisfaction, self-esteem, and competence memory (Jongman-Sereno, 2017). Attention, learning, creativity, charisma, leadership and productivity are also positively correlated to mindfulness (Langer, 2012). Positive correlations also exist between mindfulness and vision, hearing, weight loss, longevity and overall health and well-being plus other attributes (Harvard Medical School, 2008). Mindfulness negatively correlates to prejudice, burnout, accidents, stress, alcoholism, attention deficit disorders, depression, anxiety, pain and insomnia (Harvard Medical School, 2008; Jongman-Sereno, 2017; Langer, 2012). Adverse effects to mindful practices also exist.

Adverse effects.

Adverse effects of mindful meditation practices have been reported in rare cases of long-term meditators during experience of extreme meditational mental states (Shapiro, 1992). Transient negative effects have also been reported during meditation (Vanderkooi, 1997). Brown University approved Lindahl and colleagues' study on adverse effects of mindful training, which used a self-report interview process (n=25) from 2010-2016 and a Buddhist meditation intervention (2017). To qualify, participants must have had adverse reactions to Buddhist derived meditation practices prior to 2010. Their past results ranged from minimal/transient to severe/lasting adverse reactions, such as depressive states or undesirable memories. The researchers talked on the phone to participants for approximately one hour with open-ended questions about their meditation practices. The participant's experiences ranged from very positive to very negative for each person. All participant responses were considerably different. The study used seven domains of analysis: cognitive perceptual, affective, somatic, conative, sense of self, and social (Lindahl, Fisher, Cooper, Rosen, & Britton, 2017).

Risk factors found in the study were lack of sleep, inadequate diet, and lack of exercise which led to increases in destabilizing or negative meditation experiences. Recreational drug use was another risk factor for negative experiences but cited by some as helpful in negotiating negative meditative events later. Some of the subjects were hospitalized during the time frame for psychotherapy or medical treatment (Lindahl, et al., 2017). Practice approach or incorrectness of technique was also a risk factor for negative outcomes. Amount, intensity or inconsistency of practice was identified as a risk factor, too. All participants were mandated to practice one Buddhist meditation style for the study and the researchers found that the type of mindful practice can be a mismatch to the practitioner. Another risk factor is negative relationships throughout life, especially to teachers. Absent, unhelpful, not sympathetic meditation teachers and meditation community relationships predicted worse meditative difficulty vs. supportive, helpful and understanding teachers. This also held true for relationships outside their personal meditation groups (Lindahl, et al., 2017). The risk factors reported in Lindahl and colleagues study (2017) revealed that the level of well-being in their participants was poor from the beginning and throughout the study.

The most powerful risk factor of mindful programs is the quality of the mindful research being produced (Van Dam, van Vugt, Vago, Schmalzl, Saron, Olendzki, ... & Fox, 2018). In a critical study, Van Dam and colleagues (2018) found four major risk factors for mindful practices: "insufficient construct validity in research measures of mindfulness, challenges to (clinical) intervention research methodology, potential adverse effects from practicing mindfulness (referenced from: Lindahl, et al., 2017), questionable technological interpretations of data from contemplative neuroscience concerning the mental processes and brain mechanisms underlying mindfulness," (p. 42).

The Van Dam and colleagues research team argues that mindfulness measurement tools are new and have not adequately been validated. Also, questionnaires, surveys and self-reports can easily be skewed by multiple factors which can make them potentially unreliable. According to Van Dam and colleagues, multiple, large, longitudinal randomized control trials which consider participant preferences of mindfulness practices to determine the full benefits and costs are missing from the literature (2018). The researchers are not fully convinced about the reliability and even warn against neuroimage findings concerning the brain (Van Dam, et al., 2018). With the previous warning in mind, next will be the examination of mindfulness programs and the brain literature.

Brain effects.

Functional MRI's have limitations and findings can be misinterpreted due to head turning and cardio/respiratory changes creating differences between individuals (Thompson, 2017; Van Dam, et al., 2018). Brain differences make findings hard to extrapolate to groups or the population and calculating valid estimates of effect size is extremely difficult in neuroimaging data (Thompson, 2017; Van Dam, et al., 2018). Additionally, researchers recognize that collecting data in a clinical environment may cause different results when compared to a natural environment. One type of brain image cannot capture the process of mindfulness as it is not in a specific location nor is it a solitary event (Thompson, 2017). Researchers have documented size changes in areas of the brain, though.

Brain networks.

The complex resting brain state is called the default mode network (DMN). The DMN controls self-referential introspective states (Mak, Minuzzi, MacQueen, Hall, Kennedy, & Milev, 2017), among the other constructs explained here. The DMN increases connectivity to attention networks during mediation tasks (King, Angstadt, Sripada, & Liberzon, 2017) and cognitive functioning is positively correlated to DMN connectivity (Mak, et al., 2017). A meta-analysis study found the functional connectivity strength of a normal DMN follows an inverse U-shape (Mak, et al., 2017). For example, DMN connectivity is strongest during adulthood and weakest during childhood and elderly years (Mak, et al., 2017).

In a meditation study, researchers found that default mode network (DMN) brain areas are similar to meditation activity areas (Jang, Jung, Kang, Byun, Kwon, Choi, & Kwon, 2011). They compared 35 mediation practitioners with 33 non-meditators. Meditators had greater functional connectivity with the DMN in the medial prefrontal cortex area than the non-meditators did. Their findings imply that long-term meditators may be associated with functional regional brain changes for areas related to internalized attention when not meditating, as well (Jang, et al., 2011). During a study using Mindful-Based Exposure Therapy (n=31) found increased whole brain connectivity between the default mode network, functional connectivity and the dorsal attention network during the mindfulness task (King, Angstadt, Sripada, & Liberzon, 2017) using neuroimaging with a functional magnetic resonance imaging (fMRI).

Brain neuroimaging.

Neuroimaging can show where mindfulness activities land within the brain networks which can lead to associations. King and colleagues (2017) DMN network findings support mindfulness training is associated with improvements in rumination, post-traumatic stress disorder and depression. Several important studies have established beneficial outcomes like achievement of different fine motor skills, playing a musical instrument, enhanced ability for physical activities follow brain structural increases in gray and white matter (Fox, et al., 2014).

Typical brain shrinkage due to aging may be reduced in mindful practitioners (e.g., Harvard Medical School, 2008). In one study, 51-year-old mindful practitioners had equal brain gray-matter (neurons-communication) and white-matter (myelination-speed, accuracy) volume as 25-year-olds, which indicated a much slower brain decline than normal brain aging (Harvard Medical School, 2008). Gray matter concentration changes in the Mindfulness-Based Stress Reduction program (MBSR) using an fMRI measured 16 healthy non-meditators before and after an 8-week MBSR program compared with a 17-person waitlist group (Hölzel, Carmody, Vangel, Congleton, Yerramsetti, Gard, & Lazar, 2011). Increases in grey matter were confirmed for the intervention group in the left hippocampus, posterior cingulate cortex, temporo-parietal junction and the cerebellum suggesting gray matter concentration increases in brain areas involving learning, memory processes, emotion regulation, self-referential processing and perspective taking (Hölzel, et al., 2011). Additional measurable brain changes with mindful practices include, enlargement of the hippocampus (learning and memory), enlargement of the insula (convergent information processor), a shrinking amygdala (anxiety, fear, stress), improvements in the temporo-parietal junction (empathy) and improved changes in the brain stem mood molecules (Harvard Medical School, 2008). An abnormally functioning amygdala has been associated with anxiety, depression and post-traumatic stress disorder (Shin, & Liberzon, 2010).

In a meta-analysis using 22 neuroimaging studies comparing novice (n=11) vs. experienced meditators (n=12), researchers documented a difference (Falcone, & Jerram, 2018). For novices, the focus of brain activity appears to be in the insula. Experienced meditators show their foci of brain activity in the frontal gyrus and the globus pallidus (Falcone, & Jerram, 2018). A systematic review of seven fMRI studies also found a focus of activity in the insula but they could not find robust evidence for the prefrontal cortex sub-regions (Young, van der Velden, Craske, Pallesen, Fjorback, Roepstorff, & Parsons, 2017). Another fMRI meta-analysis using 78 studies and a total of 527 meditation participants found medium effect sizes for activation and deactivation consistently in the insula, pre-supplementary motor cortices, dorsal anterior cingulate cortex and the fronto-polar cortex during seven different types of meditation practices: visualization, sense-withdrawal, non-dual awareness practices, focused attention, mantra recitation, open monitoring and compassion/loving-kindness (Fox, Dixon, Nijeboer, Girn, Floman, Lifshitz, ... & Christoff, 2016). Another meta-analysis using 21 neuroimaging studies totaling 300 meditation practitioners found a global medium effect size for eight consistent brain areas altered and increased in meditators: the frontopolar cortex/BA 10 (key to meta-awareness), sensory cortices and insula (exteroceptive and interoceptive body awareness), hippocampus (memory consolidation and reconsolidation), anterior and mid cingulate/orbitofrontal cortex (self and emotion regulation) and superior longitudinal fasciculus; corpus callosum (intra and inter hemispheric communication), (Fox, Nijeboer, Dixon, Floman, Ellamil, Rumak, . . . & Christoff, 2014).

A specific fMRI study of mindful meditation-chanting compared the "OM" chant to and "SSSS" chant in 12 healthy men, with 10 rounds of 15 second on/off chanting and found a significant deactivation of the anterior cingulate, para-hippocampal gyri, thalami, hippocampi, bilateral orbitofrontal and the right amygdala in comparison to the brain resting state, only during the "OM" chant. (Kalyani, Bangalore, Venkatasubramanian, Ganesan, Arasappa, Rashmi, ... & Gangadhar, 2011). The following table outlines where these neuroimaging studies found brain activity during meditation and why type of meditation was done with whom.

Table 1. Chart of neuroimaging brain activity during meditation

Meditation Activity location	Population	Type of Meditation
Insula	Novices (Falcone, & Jerram, 2018); Mean age = 30, possibly novice participants due to age (Young, et al., 2017); experienced meditators (Fox, et al., 2016); Global medium effect size, 20-65 years old, structural increase changes (Fox, et al., 2014)	Various mindful meditations (Falcone, & Jerram, 2018); MBCT mindfulness based cognitive therapy, MBSR mindfulness based stress reduction (Young, et al., 2017); See below for (Fox, et al., 2016) and (Fox, et al., 2014)
Frontal gyrus & globus pallidus	Experienced meditators (Falcone, & Jerram, 2018);	Various mindful meditations (Falcone, & Jerram, 2018)

Pre-supplementary motor cortices, dorsal anterior cingulate cortex and the fronto-polar cortex	Global medium effect size, experienced meditators (Fox, et al., 2016); Global medium effect size, age 20-65, structural increase changes (Fox, et al., 2014)	Focused attention meditation, mantra meditation, open monitoring attention meditation, loving kindness meditation (Fox, et al., 2016); See below for (Fox, et al., 2014)
Sensory cortices, hippocampus, and superior longitudinal fasciculus; corpus callosum	Global medium effect size, age 20-65 structural increase changes (Fox, et al., 2014)	Insight, Zen, Tibetan Buddhist, MBSR; mindfulness-based stress reduction, IBMT; integrative body-mind training, BWV; brain wave vibration, Soham, LKM; loving kindness meditation, various meditations (Fox, et al., 2014)
Deactivation of the anterior cingulate, para-hippocampal gyri, thalami, hippocampi, bilateral orbitofrontal and the right amygdala in comparison to the brain resting state	Age 22-39, n=12, 4 = experienced, 8 − novices (Kalyani, et al., 2011)	OM chant

There are clearly documented changes in the brain with mindful programs but do those changes affect the physical health of PT patients enough to validate using mindful interventions?

Physical health effects.

According to a lecture by Harvard Medical School, cell production improves and positive changes in gene expression occur after mindful practices (2008). Enhanced gene-energy metabolism, mitochondria function, insulin secretion and telomere maintenance (age control) are all improved with mindful awareness practice (Harvard Medical School, 2008). After Eight weeks of a 20-minute mindful practice inflammation reduction genes turned on, plus immune system changes occurred (Harvard Medical School, 2008). This is important because the immune system plays a central role in physical health.

Immune system.

The immune system protects the body from disease and detrimental foreign bodies (Zimmerman, 2016). The immune system is capable of identifying and resolving attacks by viruses, bacteria, parasites, cancers and additional threats (Zimmerman, 2016). The immune system fluctuates in strength and capabilities according to the autonomic nervous system (Diego, Field, Sanders, & Hernandez-Reif, 2004).

Key players for the immune system are human natural killer cells which "eat" cancer, bacteria and virus cells. Cortisol, a hormone increased by the sympathetic nervous system (SNS), "eats" natural killer cells belonging to the immune system. An indicator of increased SNS activity is low tone vagal activity as discussed in the *Psychological health effects* section of this paper. Thus, low tone vagal activity (SNS) indirectly lowers the amount of natural killer cells fighting for the immune system (Diego, Field, Sanders, & Hernandez-Reif, M.,2004; Brittenden,

Heys, Ross, & Eremin, 1996). Low vagal tone also forecasts high inflammation (Thayer & Sternberg, 2006), myocardial infarction risk and lower survival odds after heart failure among other poor health outcomes (Bibevski & Dunlap, 2011).

A research study (Kok, Coffey, Cohn, Catalino, Vacharkulksemsuk, Algoe, ... & Fredrickson, 2013), took advantage of measurable vagal tone outputs for its quantifiable outcomes. To measure vagal tone, high-frequency components (0.12-0.4 Hz) of the heart rate signal reflect vagal influences on the heart. Even though vagal nerve tone fluctuates with the nervous system (PNS/SNS input) its baseline, the constant input to keep the automatic organs like the heart running, was once considered stable and unchanging. Vagal nerve baseline is now known to be changeable and possess plastic properties (Kok, et al., 2013). If one's vagal baseline was lower than average, that individual would constantly present as a person with more "fight or flight" (SNS) characteristics and most probably poorer physical health due to the reasons explained previously concerning the SNS. Next is an example of this phenomenon.

Researchers used 71 university faculty/staff and one intervention to test the baseline of the vagus nerve (Kok, et al., 2013). For six weeks, subjects performed a mandatory one-hour per week loving-kindness meditation. In addition, they self-decided frequency and duration of daily meditations. Baseline vagal nerve tone was taken two weeks before the intervention and one week after. The baseline vagal tone was higher post intervention with variations. The amount of increase in vagal tone post intervention positively correlated to the increased amount of self-reported positive emotion and positive social connections experienced by the end of the study. For participants who started with a higher baseline vagal tone, their positive emotions had a steeper increase during the study. (Kok, et al., 2013). Increasing vagus nerve tone and positive social engagement are reciprocally influenced by self-generated positive emotion, as in the Kok study (2013). Additional research exists for different types of mindful interventions, other than meditation, which increase vagal tone and thus PNS input making them measurable candidates to protect physical health.

Interventions.

Mindful exercise interventions are needed to fulfill physical therapy goals but how do they compare to the previous meditation research? When participants are doing neuroimaging in an fMRI, they have to lye very still making meditation the mindful intervention of choice to study for neuroimaging. Also, meditation is very simple to administer during a research study but all mindful interventions have a lot in common. They are under the same umbrella of mindful because they all require the elements described in the *Mindful Definitions* section of this paper. Mindful exercises just add body movements to this meditative process, so they have additional properties not different ones.

Three mindful interventions show great promise: yoga, tai chi and massage therapy (Riley & Park, 2015). Massage therapy is equivalent to manual therapy which is already in use, has very good outcomes and is billable by PTs. Let's look at yoga exercises.

In a systematic review of 71 journal articles (Riley & Park, 2015), yoga improved positive affect, mindfulness and self-compassion with inhibition in the posterior hypothalamus, decreased interleukin-6 (inflammation indicator), decreased C-reactive protein and decreased cortisol levels. Yoga also raises vagal tone (Sullivan, Erb, Schmalzl, Moonaz, Noggle, ... & Taylor 2018) as does massage therapy (Hernandez-Reif, Field, Ironson, Beutler, Vera, Hurley, ... & Hernandez-Reif, M., 2005; Hernandez-Reif, Ironson, Field, Hurley, Katz, Diego, ... & Burman, I., 2004). Research on tai chi shows high tone vagal activity, as well (Wei, Li, Yue, Ma, Chang, Yi, ... & Zuo, 2016).

Each intervention requires different senses which means different brain processing pathways are activated and strengthened to achieve high vagal tone (Kayser & Shams, 2015). For example, yoga and tai chi require muscle movement, balance and eyesight brain processes. Sitting meditations and massage do not. Breath regulation, which directly affects the vagus nerve (Song, Liu, Proctor, & Yu, 2015), is required by all four interventions but at different tempos and efforts requiring different neuro-pathways (Kayser & Shams, 2015). Yoga and massage researchers hypothesize the increase in vagal tone comes from pressure on the skin receptors (also part of the vagus nerve system) unlike tai chi and meditation (Hernandez-Reif, 2004; Hernandez-Reif, 2005). Both yoga and qigong (tai chi) decrease anxiety, depression and sleep disorders (Field, Diego, Delgado, & Medina, 2013;Tsang, Chan, & Cheung, 2008). A literature review compiling yoga journal articles, reports that yoga improves job stress, anxiety, depression, sleep, low back pain, headaches, osteoarthritis, rheumatoid arthritis, coronary artery disease, hypertension, autoimmune conditions, asthma, diabetes, multiple sclerosis, lymphoma, breast cancer, hypertension and preterm labor, stress, labor pain, heartrate and blood pressure, pulmonary measures, weight loss, balance, flexibility and strength (Field, 2011). Fields (2011) review sites eight problem areas in the articles concerned with participants and methods. Even though Fields (2011) is concerned, there are multiple articles in the literature that defend this stance on the effects of yoga. Combining the four interventions of yoga, meditation, massage therapy and tai chi may have cumulative health benefits due to their differences, though little research on this topic has been found.

Table 2. Effects of Mindful Interventions

	Yoga	Tai Chi or Qigong	Massage	Meditation
increases	**increases**	**increases**	**increases**	**increases**
positive affect, mindfulness and self-compassion	(Riley & Park, 2015)	**No change** (Lee, Harvey, Wong, Price, Han, Chung,... & Wang, 2017)	(Maratos, Duarte, Barnes, McEwan, Sheffield, & Gilbert, 2017)	(Jongman-Sereno, K. 2017)
vagal tone (parasympathetic nervous system-PNS activation)	(Sullivan, Erb, Schmalzl, Moonaz, Noggle, ... & Taylor 2018)	(Wei, Li, Yue, Ma, Chang, Yi, ... & Zuo, 2016)	(Hernandez-Reif, Field, Ironson, Beutler, Vera, Hurley, ... & Hernandez-Reif, M., 2005; Hernandez-(Reif, Ironson, Field, Hurley, Katz, Diego, ... & Burman, I., 2004)	(Kok, Coffey, Cohn, Catalino, Vacharkulksemsuk, Algoe, ... & Fredrickson, 2013)
skin receptor input for vagal tone	(Hernandez-Reif, 2004; Hernandez-Reif, 2005)	x	(Hernandez-Reif, 2004; Hernandez-Reif, 2005)	x
muscle movement, balance, strength, flexibility	(Guleria, Arora, Mohan, Kumar, & Kumar, 2015; Field, 2011)-literature review	(Zou, Wang, Xiao, Fang, Zhang, Li,... & Liu, 2017).-systematic review	Chatchawan, Eungpinichpong, Plandee, & Yamauchi, 2015).	x

pulmonary (breathing) improvements	**Strong** (Guleria, Arora, Mohan, Kumar, & Kumar, 2015; Field, 2011) literature review	**Modest** (Ng, L., Chiang, Tang, Siu, Fung, Lee, & Tam, 2014).	x	x
immune system function	(Field, 2011) literature review	(Zeng, Luo, Xie, Huang, & Cheng, 2014)- meta-analysis	(Tejero-Fernández, Membrilla-Mesa, Galiano-Castillo, & Arroyo-Morales, 2015)	(Schilling, R. 2017)
quality of life	**children** (Bazzano, Anderson, Hylton, & Gustat, 2018), **Adults** (Guleria, Arora, Mohan, Kumar, & Kumar, 2015)	(Zou, Wang, Xiao, Fang, Zhang, Li,... & Liu, 2017).- systematic review	(Yuan, Matsutani, & Marques, 2015)- systematic review	significant effects (Hilton, Hempel, Ewing, Apaydin, Xenakis, Newberry,... & Maglione, 2016) systematic review with meta-analysis, significant
decreases	**decreases**	**decreases**	**decreases**	**decreases**
posterior hypothalamus , interleukin-6 (inflammation indicator), C-reactive protein	(Guleria, Arora, Mohan, Kumar, & Kumar, 2015; Riley & Park, 2015)	**No change** (Campo, Light, O'Connor, Nakamura, Lipschitz, LaStayo, ... & Martins, 2015)	**Significant** Dupuy, Douzi, Theurot, Bosquet, & Dugué, 2018). meta-analysis	(Schilling, R. 2017)
cortisol levels	(Field, 2011) literature review	(Campo, Light, O'Connor, Nakamura, Lipschitz, LaStayo, ... & Martins, 2015; Zeng, Luo, Xie, Huang, & Cheng, 2014)- meta-analysis	(Maratos, Duarte, Barnes, McEwan, Sheffield, & Gilbert, 2017)	in children (Yoo, Lee, Lee, Shin, Park, Yoon, & Yu, 2016); in adults (Fan, Tang, & Posner, 2014).

anxiety, depression, sleep disorders (fatigue)	(Field, Diego, Delgado, & Medina, 2013; Tsang, Chan, & Cheung, 2008)	(Field, Diego, Delgado, & Medina, 2013; Tsang, Chan, & Cheung, 2008; Zeng, Luo, Xie, Huang, & Cheng, 2014)- meta-analysis	medium effects (Yuan, Matsutani, & Marques, 2015)- systematic review (Dupuy, Douzi, Theurot, Bosquet, & Dugué, 2018). meta-analysis	significant effects (Hilton, Hempel, Ewing, Apaydin, Xenakis, Newberry,... & Maglione, 2016) systematic review with meta-analysis; in children (Yoo, Lee, Lee, Shin, Park, Yoon, & Yu, 2016).
pain, musculoskeletal disorders	(Guleria, Arora, Mohan, Kumar, & Kumar, 2015; Field, 2011) literature review	(Hall, Copsey, Richmond, Thompson, Ferreira, Latimer, & Maher, 2017)- meta-analysis (Lee, Harvey, Wong, Price, Han, Chung,... & Wang, 2017)	significant effects (Yuan, Matsutani, & Marques, 2015). systematic review	small effects for chronic pain (Hilton, Hempel, Ewing, Apaydin, Xenakis, Newberry,... & Maglione, 2016) systematic review with meta-analysis; significant effects (Zeidan, Emerson, Farris, Ray, Jung, Y., McHaffie, & Coghill, 2015).
resting heart rate, high blood pressure	(Field, 2011) literature review	(Campo, Light, O'Connor, Nakamura, Lipschitz, LaStayo, ... & Martins, 2015)	(Nelson, 2015).	(Bai, Chang, Chen, Yang, & Chi, 2015). systematic review with meat-analysis

PT scope of practice categories	Yoga	Tai Chi or Qigong	Massage	Meditation
Musculoskeletal	x	x	x	
Neuromuscular	x	x	x	

Cardiovascular/pulmonary	x	x	x	x
Integumentary disorders	x	x	x	x
Pain	x	x	x	x

Although massage or manual therapy does show results for decreasing pain, a meta-analysis of seven articles out of 1169 found were used to analyze improvements of manual therapy added to exercise physical therapy treatments for the neck. Interestingly, the addition of manual therapy plus exercise had the same results as exercise alone (Fredin, K., & Lorås, H. (2017). Manual therapy may not be necessary in neck treatments if the best practice exercises are used.

The key to finding more positively influential interventions may be to look at what the known interventions all have in common and then find similarly structured interventions. All four require the combination of the mind fixated in the present, body movement attention (either in controlled patterns or stillness) and breath regulation (whether high or low).

Few interventions match these criteria. Sports taught with a high level of mindfulness might qualify. American coaches and trainers would need to change their styles from win and push harder to focus intensely, regulate intensely, and recover frequently to a peaceful (PNS) state. The highest level athletes discover 'the zone' of focus and regulation on their own but most sports do not coach the previous approach. Yoga, meditation and tai chi are simple, adaptable and can be free. Minimal space, no equipment, no special floors, no shoes and no supervision are required, making them a reasonable intervention choice to support 1. positive emotions and affect, 2. high vagal tone and 3. perceived positive social connections, as described previously in Porges's Polyvagal Theory.

In contrast, exercise interventions like aerobics and weight lifting require activation of the SNS to increase heart rate. So, low vagal tone, which indicates activation of the SNS, is associated with exercise and stress (Lucas, Heidi, Porges, & Rejeski, 2016). Even in rigorous yoga and tai chi exercises the nervous system alternates from SNS to PNS activation promoting efficient shifting from arousal to calm (Lucas, et al., 2016) leaving the practitioner with a higher vagal tone baseline post intervention (Sullivan, Erb, Schmalzl, Moonaz, Noggle, Taylor, Porges, & Porges, 2018). Autonomic neural regulation, the ability to change from SNS to PNS activation reciprocally, is linked to improved breast and prostate cancer outcomes (Couck, Marechal, Moorthamers, Laethem, & Gidron, 2016; Magnon, Hall, Lin, et al., 2013). This evidence shows the effects for patients but healthcare workers using mindful programs have effects from the interventions as well.

Staff effects.

In 2018, researchers Duggan and Julliard conducted a multi-level, hospital staff, mindful education research study with social workers and therapists (n=4), nurses (n=7), doctors (n=2) and administrative staff and leaders (n=7) as leadership facilitators. The healthcare facilities used were one inner-city teaching hospital, a number of schools, public clinics, a homeless-persons' clinic and diverse social support centers. All 20 volunteered to educate their respective departments (Duggan, & Julliard, 2018). Due to hospital time constraints the obvious choice for a starting point was a brief intervention (Duggan, & Julliard, 2018). The Mindful Minute Intervention (MMI), a brief one to three-minute staff intervention based on the *Joy of Living* program of the Tergarr Meditation Community, was used. Focused attention, open presence and a relaxed recognition of awareness was central to the practice incorporating awareness and concentration (Duggan, & Julliard, 2018).

The volunteer facilitators were asked to begin meetings, shifts, patient room-entry and/or classes with MMI and were interviewed post experiment, six weeks later. Facilitators were taught the guidelines of how to introduce the MMI to a group, when it should be used and how to lead the MMI. Training included an in-person one-hour group training with role-play/feedback and a 10-minute online training video. A printed guide and script were provided for both the one minute and three-minute options. Predicted obstacles for facilitators were coercion refusal, 'is it my place' type questioning, burden of leadership and competing priorities (Duggan, & Julliard, 2018).

Six weeks later, facilitators reported staff benefits which included personal stress relief, positive energy shift, increased level/tenor of group participation, improved sense of human connection, caring and shared reality, positive-tone foundation for the segment of time (i.e. meeting), increased personal focus for reduction of errors, better productivity/efficiency, increased presence with a quality of non-resistance to current circumstances, desire for more healthy self-care, immediate emotional presence benefit and relaxation of the practitioner contributing to relaxation of the patient (Duggan, & Julliard, 2018). The researchers predicted all the outcomes from their preliminary research but in a different frequency amount order than expected. The only two outcomes they did not predict at all were energy shift and improved sense of human connection. Surprisingly to Duggan and Julliard (2018), both energy shift and improved sense of human connection scored in the top four for most frequently occurring. The researchers were also surprised by the high number of interpersonal attributes (three of the top five) compared to intrapersonal attributes (Duggan, & Julliard, 2018). In contrast to this one study for hospital staff, many studies have been conducted with healthcare students which could be generalizable.

Finally, a meta-analysis of 19 studies of students (grand total of participants, n =1,815) in the fields of medicine (n=10), nursing (n=4), psychiatry (n=1), social work (n=1) and other healthcare realms (n=3) analyzed the effects of mindfulness training for healthcare students' mood, stress, depression, self-efficacy, empathy and anxiety (McConville, McAleer, & Hahne, 2017). Results showed decreases in stress, anxiety and depression along with improvements for mindfulness, mood, self-efficacy and empathy post mindful interventions. This meta-analysis recommended mindful training be implemented into the training of healthcare professionals due to its easy implementation and positive results (McConville, McAleer, & Hahne, 2017).

Staff buy-in.

Leadership buy-in is a program risk factor for program failure (Byron, et al., 2015). Two of the previous strong and current systematic reviews conducted by Barnes and colleagues (2018) and Mileski and colleagues (2017), link decreasing hospital profits with poor quality care and improving hospital patient care with staff training as the evidence-based, best-practice option. These studies show that it is in every healthcare facility's financial best interest to invest in the mental health of their staff.

Also important to healthcare is the accessibility of a comprehensive, evidence-based, time-efficient, cost-effective mindful program that their staff will accept. According to Byron and colleagues (2015), successful buy-in for staff requires slow implementation with volunteers which helps accommodate fear of the unknown or fear of change. Best-practice would be to introduce the mindfulness cultural change in phases with the six-week MMI (e.g., Byron, et al., 2015; Duggan, & Julliard, 2018) as Phase I.

Research claims mindful programs are more successful in the presence of local champions, leadership buy-in, prior mindfulness exposure of participants and if the program was voluntary vs. mandatory (Byron, Aiedonis, McGrath, Frazier, deTorrijos, & Fulwiler, 2015). In contrast, downfalls to successful programs are insufficient training coverage, insufficient time given to planning and effective program communication, not enough time for staff attendance to training sessions and logistics (Byron, et al., 2015).

Play-Oriented Functional Activities as Interventions

Many of the recent journal articles written concerning play and seniors are about seniors using video games during their physical therapy treatments. These articles show positive outcomes for postural control, gait and cardiorespiratory fitness when compared to conventional physical therapy (Bacha, Gomes, de Freitas, Viveiro, da Silva, Bueno,... & D'Andrea Greve, 2018; Hossain, Rahman, & Muhammad, 2017). A meta-analysis of 18 randomized controlled trials (n=765) found that the use of exercise-based, active video games (AVGs) resulted in the researchers concluding AVGs were more effective than conventional physical therapy exercise or no treatment for mobility and balance in seniors (Taylor, Kerse, Frakking, & Maddison, 2018). A review of the neuroimaging literature supports improvements in executive functioning of cognitive processes for AVGs, as well (Rose Ru-Whui, Sung, & Chang, 2013). One of the studies in the review specifically investigated people age 60-73 (Van Muijden, Band, & Hommel, 2012). After gaming, this population saw neuroimaging improvements in cognitive control function in inhibition attention, inductive reasoning, and selective attention (Van Muijden, Band, & Hommel, 2012). None of these articles discussed if it was the playing element that produced the positive outcomes.

No current play specific functional activity journal articles were found for the senior population but they may exist. The benefits of play has been deeply studied in children and due to neuroimaging finding that the brain is plastic at any age, these findings may be generalizable to seniors (Volkman, 2018). Researchers Singer and colleagues (2006) found that play not only motivates learning but it enhances it. Cognitive and social-emotional growth also result from play activities (Singer, Golinkoff, & Hirsh-Pasek, 2006). Education and learning is a primary goal for patients in physical therapy. Patient education is a timed insurance code billable by PTs for the benefit of improving patient outcomes. Play is a valuable tool that many times goes unused by PTs during their serious exercise drills.

Functional physical therapy activities like getting off of the floor, reaching, grasping, walking fast and moving from sitting to standing are movements required of play. Thus, play with functional activity physical therapy goals are a good fit.

Intergenerational Care

Zoos individually caged monkeys, tigers and bears for centuries. In the past 20 years, animal caregivers at zoos researched and replaced the outdated cage model with a habitat model for improved psychological and physical animal health (Rose & Croft, 2015, p. 123). In the habitat model, the monkeys live all together on a large piece of property and their caregivers and healthcare providers come to them, on their natural turf.

American geriatric and pre-school populations suffer in age-segregated captivity like the old-style zoo monkeys, tigers and bears. According to a journal article in *The Science in the Service of Animal Welfare* (Rose & Croft, 2015, p. 123), "Disruption to social bonds may lead to impoverished welfare and stress to individuals which have seen their social support compromised." Like the monkeys, both geriatrics and preschoolers are given a minimal amount of choice about the cage they live in and who resides with them. Caregivers make those decisions.

Inter-generational care and social living, generally, increases social stress. Even though stress is usually interpreted as negative, two animal studies argue the opposite. The studies proclaim the goal of animal husbandry is to create conditions that enable a full range of behavior repertoire which include arousal and stress (Chamove & Anderson, 1989; Moodie & Chamove, 1990). Animal social living and its potential problems and complexity have been linked to the evolution of intelligence (Byrne & Whiten, 1988; Dunbar & Shultz, 2007; Psquaretta et al., 2014). Due to these animal studies, it is commonplace in zoos to provide challenging, complex social and physical environments (Buchanan-smith, Griciute, Daoudi, Leonardi, & Whiten,

2013; Hardie, 1997; Leonardi Buchanan-Smith, Dufour, Macdonald, & Whiten, 2011'
MacDonald & Whiten, 2011; Sodaro, 1999; Veasey & Jammer, 2010). The conclusion of the
animal kingdom evidence points to, "Primate well-being is not so much a function of
confinement as of the presence of relevant incentives to engage in species-appropriate behavior"
(Chang, Forthman, Maple, 1999). Universally, humans have lived in inter-generational clans
throughout time until the last century with the onslaught of daycare centers and nursing homes.

Although not well known and not yet popular, intergenerational care has been researched
since the 1990's. Even the government site of the Commission on Affordable Housing and
Health Facility Needs for Seniors in the 21st Century received and listed a report on June 28,
2002 about intergenerational care benefits (2002).

Definition of terms.

The intergenerational care concept consists of seniors and preschool aged children.
Preschoolers are chosen because they can interact verbally and physically with the senior yet
they do not have to adhere to the daily demands of school, yet. Some intergenerational care units
are mixing seniors with developmentally delayed children of many ages and the seniors are
participating in their caregiving needs and activities (AARP, 2018). Proposals are currently being
submitted for school based programs with seniors as mentors (AARP, 2018). Many groups are
springing up around this concept: Generations United, Center for Intergenerational Practice and
the Journal of Intergenerational Relationships (DeVore, Winchell, & Rowe, 2016). St. Ann
Center for Intergenerational Care in Milwaukee, Wisconsin and the Intergenerational Center for

Learning by Providence Health in Seattle, Washington are the two of the most prominent facilities in America, both are Catholic non-profits. Many of the intergenerational programs are sponsored by a church as is Bethlehem Intergenerational Center in Grand Rapids, Michigan (Lutheran). It is difficult to know exactly how many exist and in what form but according to Generations United (AARP, 2018) facilities are scarce but most states have at least one.

Seniors' physical health effects.

According to Flora and Faulkner (2006), there is very little in the literature about the physical benefits of intergenerational care. After a review of the literature Flora and Faulner (2006) only found four articles that took physical measurements of the seniors. Due to the limited evidence and the weak methodology used, the authors could not reach any strong conclusions (Flora, & Faulkner, 2006). They report that further research is clearly needed concerning the physical benefits of seniors in intergenerational care(Flora, & Faulkner, 2006). Even though there are very few articles on quantitative physical data, there are articles about how the psychological benefits effect physical health indirectly.

Although social connections clearly contribute to physical health (Barger, 2013; Berkman & Glass, 2000; Cohen, 2004; Holt-Lunstad, Smith, & Layton, 2010), the quality of the social relationships play an important role (Rook, August, & Sorkin, 2011). Diversity in social networks is one key element in better health outcomes as in greater immunity to infectious disease (e.g., Cohen, Doyle, Skoner, Rabin, & Gwaltney, 1997). Social relationships compares with smoking and alcohol consumption for its effect on mortality risk (Holt-Lunstad et al.,

2010). Many times seniors do not have control over their social interactions (Martire, & Franks, 2014). For instance, they may have children and grandchildren but never see them. They may have children and grandchildren around all the time but watch television in a private room and do not interact with them, depleting their relationship health benefits.

In a new intergenerational care rehab center (Bernard's Residential Care Home) backed by Dr. Zoe Wyrko (a Geriatric Medicine Consultant for University Hospitals Birmingham), National Hospital Society (NHS) Foundation Trust and Heart of England NHS Foundation Trust found that according to their employee's senior morale, motivation, happiness, and mobility increased (Ashurst, 2018). The workers noted that the senior started using multiple senses instead relying on their strongest abilities (Ashurst, 2018).

Many seniors report feeling lonely and are socially isolated. While both effect quality of life and well-being, according to Steptoe and colleagues (2013) it is social isolation that effects mortality. Social isolation is on the rise due to poor economic resources, mobility impairments and the death of their same generation friends. Mortality, cardiovascular disease, infectious illness, cognitive deterioration, high blood pressure, rising C-reactive protein and elevated fibrinogen result from social isolation in seniors (Steptoe, Shankar, Demakakos, & Wardle, 2013). When stressed, socially isolated seniors have heightened inflammatory and metabolic responses when compared to non-socially isolated seniors (Steptoe, et al., 2013).

Seniors' psychological effects.

During intergenerational care, two basic psychological effects occur throughout the literature; seniors increase active engagement in activities and present with more positive affect (Jarrott, & Bruno, 2007). Engagement is defined as positive social interactions, nonsocial-nonproductive activity and solitary productive activity (Short-DeGraff, & Diamond, 1996). Using the Intergenerational Program Quality Assessment tool, researchers found that engagement increased when both generations regularly met in a shared location, had a wide variety of choices which focused on the process (not product) and when everyone, including staff, reflected before and afterward on modifications of task (Epstein, & Boisvert, 2006). The Intergenerational Observation Scale is another standardized measurement tool that can be used (Jarrott, Smith, & Weintraub, 2008). Epstein and Boisvert (2006) also found that the seniors increased their tolerance and understanding of the younger generation. Jarrott and Bruno (2007) documented bonding between the seniors and children into close relationships and the seniors appreciated the children's diverse viewpoints about activity suggestions. As they engaged in joint activities, both the children and seniors experienced increased positive social interactions and engagement levels (Short-DeGraff, & Diamond, 1996). The seniors were also very excited to see the children each day (Ashurst, 2018).

Children's psychological effects.

The effects for children attending intergenerational care facilities includes but is not limited to: empathy and understanding for older adults, improved understanding of life cycle, overcoming misconceptions of older people and accurate knowledge about older people's contribution ability

(Devore, et al., 2016). Children in intergenerational care settings are more willing to approach older adults and share activities with them, outside the intergenerational setting (Gigliotti, Morris, Smock, Jarrott, & Graham, 2005; Gilbert & Ricketts, 2008; Hayes, 2003; Holmes, 2009)

In one study, children attended an intergenerational care program for one summer and then either agreed or disagreed with statements describing social, behavioral and physical characteristics of older adults (Aday, Sims, McDuffie, & Evans, 1996). The Children's perceptions of Aging and Elderly (CPAE) inventory was used. The children who had attended for the summer made more positive statements concerning seniors than the control group participants who did not attend, even five years after they attended the program (Aday, et al., 1996). Longevity of these positive attitude changes is seen in much of the literature. Three years after one group attended an intergenerational preschool, the children had higher levels of empathy toward seniors than children who did not attend (Femia, Zarit, Blair, Jarrott, & Bruno, 2008). In another study, children's opinions on creating a list of 17 adjective pairs describing seniors were measured against themselves; before and after intergenerational preschool. Their opinions were more positive post-attendance (Lynott, & Merola, 2007). A similar study using picture drawing had the same results showing positive improvements over the control group (Heyman, Gutheil, & White-Ryan, 2011). Child comfort levels go up and shyness goes down after intergenerational activities (Gigliotti, et al., 2005; Holmes, 2009). Three research studies (Belgrave, 2011; Middlecamp & Gross, 2002; Salari, 2002), showed no changes in children's attitudes but their methods were categorizing a child's description of the senior who needs an assistive device as a negative remark, possibly skewing their data (Femia, et al., 2008). Femia and colleagues (2008) also found that planned-activity intergenerational preschool programs produced significantly higher functioning children in social-emotional development than children who went to single generation programs.

Summary

PT's job stress has been associated with poor patient outcomes (Physical therapy workforce project, 2008). In the PT job turnover study, researchers reported that the origin of their stress is high demand plus low control but high demand plus high control is not. The solution is to raise a PTs sense of control, because lowering high demand is not an option for the job description. The literature presents this as a two-fold problem. Firstly, the current physical therapy environment model puts a PTs sense of well-being at risk. PTs (along with other healthcare workers) experience ageism, cynicism and job-burnout due to their environmental conditions leading to costly job-turnover critical to clinic patient quality care, clinic productivity, clinic sustainability and personal well-being. Secondly, PTs are knowingly under-achieving which contributes to a feeling of job burnout. Even though they know the research clearly supports a bio-psycho-social model for pain control, PTs are restricted by their scope of practice by-laws from getting paid by insurance companies for any type of psychological patient treatments. Plus, they are not trained in this area and cannot directly refer patients to mental health service. Together, physical therapy's current conditions create an unhealthy environment for not only patients to heal but for physical therapists to work in. The intergenerational research and the mindful intervention research show positive results in helping to resolve both problems while staying within a PT's scope of practice.

Mindful research supports the mind, body and brain benefits associated with improved psychological plus physical health. Using mindful interventions is billable and within the PTs scope of practice. Mindful interventions have the potential to improve a PT's sense of control over patient pain outcomes. This decreases a PT's job stress which in-turn improves patient outcomes. There is an upward spiraling effect to improving the type of intervention when it effects both the patient and the healthcare worker. The environment also contributes to the psychological component of pain. The intergenerational care research supplies an alternative supportive environment.

Most of the research on intergenerational care to date has been in analyzing the psychological benefits of both seniors and children which does have an indirect result on physical health. There is a gap in the research on quantitative research for the direct and measurable physical effects for a seniors (and children) participating in an intergenerational program (Flora and Faulkner,2006). For instance, basic physical therapy measurements like ambulation distances and quality, shoulder and knee range of motion or sit to stand capabilities were not found to report on for this literature review. The psychological effects for seniors include increased active engagement in activities, being more present with increased positive affect (Jarrott, & Bruno, 2007) and increased tolerance and understanding of the younger generation (Epstein and Boisvert, 2006). Effects for preschoolers attending intergenerational care facilities includes but is not limited to: empathy and understanding for older adults, improved understanding of life cycle, overcoming misconceptions of older people and accurate knowledge about older people's contribution ability (Devore, et al., 2016). Children in intergenerational care settings are more willing to approach older adults and share activities with them, outside the intergenerational setting (Gigliotti, Morris, Smock, Jarrott, & Graham, 2005; Gilbert & Ricketts, 2008; Hayes, 2003; Holmes, 2009)

The literature supports that pain has a psychological component and that mindful interventions have been shown to meet that need. Mindful exercises are a billable and usable intervention source for physical therapists. Although mindful interventions has a plethora of physical and neuroimaging findings to support their clinical physical therapy use, mindful intervention applications in physical therapy clinics to use as a program guide was not found but may exist in the literature.

There is a gap in the literature for an experimental medical model utilizing the assets of an intergenerational care environment couple with optimal mindful interventions which meet psychological and physical needs for geriatric physical therapy. According to this literature review appropriate interventions would include:

(a) Yoga, meditation, tai chi and self-massage of neck, feet and hands.

(b) Functional activities of daily living with a parameter of fulfillment of self-actualization strategies listed below. For example, setting realistic goals (a.) for walking distances and then patient reflecting (a. metacognition) on what one would realistically need to do to increase the distance.

(c) Activities which support any of the self-actualization strategies below. For example, all books

in the facility will contain age appropriate subject matter of (f.) in order to qualify for the

model's curriculum:

a. Think consciously about the future (set realistic goals, metacognition, etc.)

b. Introspect on inner states (mindful practices, positive psychology, etc.)

c. Observe and evaluate personal characteristics (self-empathy, self-compassion, reality checks, therapy, group therapy, mindful practices, etc.)

d. Imagine how we are perceived by others (other and self-empathy, reality checks, etc.)

e. Engage in volitional self-change (therapy, behavior modification strategies, effort, etc.)

f. Be a good consumer of psychological science (learn more about psychology research findings, religions, ancient psychology, philosophy, etc.) (Jongman-Sereno, 2017)

References

AARP (2018). America's best intergenerational communities. *Generations United.* Downloaded

5 July 2018 from https://www.aarp.org/content/dam/aarp/livable-

communities/learn/civic/americas-best-intergenerational-communities-aarp.pdf

Aday, R., Sims, C. R., McDuffie, W., & Evans, E. (1996). Changing children's attitudes toward

the elderly: The longitudinal effects of an intergenerational partners program. *Journal of*

Research in Childhood Education, 10(2), 143-151.

Allen, A. B., & Leary, M. R. (2010). Self-compassion, stress, and coping. Social and Personality

Psychology Compass, 4(2), 107–118.

American Medical Association. Code of Medical Ethics: Principle 1 2001. Downloaded 26 June

2018 from *http://www.ama-assn.org/ama/pub/physician-resources/medical-ethics/code-*

medical-ethics/principles-medical-ethics.page

American Physical Therapy Association (2011). Today's PT: a comprehensive review of 21st-

century health care profession. *APTA.* Downloaded 5 July 2018 from

https://www.apta.org/uploadedFiles/APTAorg/Practice_and_Patient_Care/PR_and_Mar

keting/Market_to_Professionals/TodaysPhysicalTherapist.pdf

American Physical Therapy Association (2018). Vision statement for the physical therapy

profession and guiding principles to achieve the vision. *APTA.* Downloaded 5 July 2018

from http://www.apta.org/Vision/

Anderson, E. Z., Gould-Fogerite, S., Pratt, C., & Perlman, A. (2015). Identifying stress and

burnout in PTs. *Physiotherapy, 101*, e1712-e1713.

Ashurst, A. (2018). How intergenerational care generates happiness. *Nursing And Residential Care, 20*(5), 234-236.

Bacha, J. M. R., Gomes, G. C. V., de Freitas, T. B., Viveiro, L. A. P., da Silva, K. G., Bueno, G. C., ... & D'Andrea Greve, J. M. (2018). Effects of Kinect adventures games versus conventional physical therapy on postural control in elderly people: a randomized controlled trial. *Games for health journal, 7*(1), 24-36.

Bai, Z., Chang, J., Chen, C., Li, P., Yang, K., & Chi, I. (2015). Investigating the effect of transcendental meditation on blood pressure: a systematic review and meta-analysis. *Journal of human hypertension, 29*(11), 653.

Bandura, A., Pastorelli, C., Barbaranelli, C., & Caprara, G. V. (1999). Self-efficacy pathways to childhood depression. *Journal of Personality and social Psychology, 76*(2), 258.

Barger, S. D. (2013). Social integration, social support and mortality in the US National Health Interview Survey. *Psychosomatic Medicine, 75,* 510–517.

Bazzano, A. N., Anderson, C. E., Hylton, C., & Gustat, J. (2018). Effect of mindfulness and yoga on quality of life for elementary school students and teachers: results of a randomized controlled school-based study. *Psychology Research and Behavior Management, 11,* 81.

Beaumont, E., Irons, C., Rayner, G., & Dagnall, N. (2016b). Does compassion focused therapy training for health care educators and providers increase self-compassion and reduce self-persecution and self-criticism? *Journal of Continuing Education in the Health Professions, 36(*1), 4–10.

Belgrave, M. (2011). The effect of a music therapy intergenerational program on children and

older adults' intergenerational interactions, cross-age attitudes, and older adults'

psychosocial well-being. *Journal of Music Therapy, 48*(4), 486-508.

Berkman, L. F., & Glass, T. (2000). Social integration, social networks, social support, and

health. In L. F. Berkman & I. Kawachi (Eds.), *Social epidemiology* (pp. 137–173). New

York, NY: Oxford University Press.

Bibevski, S., & Dunlap, M. E. (2011). Evidence for impaired vagus nerve activity in heart

failure. *Heart Failure Reviews*, *16,* 129–135.

Bodner, E. (2009). On the origins of ageism among older and younger adults. *International*

Psycho-

Boersma, K., & Lindblom, K. (2009). Stability and change in burnout profiles over time: a

prospective study in the working population. *Work & Stress 23*, 264–283.

Brittenden, J., Heys, S. D., Ross, J., & Eremin, O. (1996). Natural killer cells and

cancer. *Cancer*, *77*(7), 1226-1243.

Brown, K. W., Ryan, R. M., & Creswell, J. D. (2007). Mindfulness: Theoretical foundations and

evidence for its salutary effects. *Psychological Inquiry*, *18*(4), 211-237.

Buchanan-Smith, H. M., Griciute, J., Daoudi, S., Leonardi, R., & Whiten, A. (2013).

Interspecific interactions and welfare implications in mixed species communities of

capuchin (Sapajus apella) and squirrel monkeys (Saimiri sciureus) over 3 years. Applied

Animal Behaviour Science, 147, 324–333.

Bureau of Labor and Statistics (2018). Occupational outlook handbook: PTs. *Government Agency*. Downloaded on 5 July 2018 from *https://www.bls.gov/ooh/healthcare/physical-therapists.htm*

Byrne, R. W., & Whiten, A. (1988). Machiavellian intelligence: Social expertise and the evolution of intellect in monkeys, apes and humans. Oxford, UK: Clarendon Press

Byron, G., Ziedonis, D. M., McGrath, C., Frazier, J. A., & Fulwiler, C. (2015). Implementation of mindfulness training for mental health staff: Organizational context and stakeholder perspectives. *Mindfulness, 6*(4), 861-872.

Calder Calisi, C. (2017). The effects of the relaxation response on nurses' level of anxiety, depression, well-being, work-related stress, and confidence to teach patients. *Journal of Holistic Nursing, 35*(4), 318-327.

Campo, M. A., Weiser, S., & Koenig, K. L. (2009). Job strain in PTs. *Physical therapy, 89*(9), 946-956.

Campo, R. A., Light, K. C., O'Connor, K., Nakamura, Y., Lipschitz, D., LaStayo, P. C., ... & Martins, T. B. (2015). Blood pressure, salivary cortisol, and inflammatory cytokine outcomes in senior female cancer survivors enrolled in a tai chi randomized controlled trial. *Journal of Cancer Survivorship, 9*(1), 115-125.

Canadian Nurses Association (2009). Tested solutions for eliminating Canada's registered nurse shortage. Ottawa, Canada: *Canadian Nurses Association*. Downloaded 4 April 2018 from *https://www.cna-aiic.ca/en/news-room/news-releases/2009/eliminating-canadas-rn-shortage*

Canadian Nurses Association (2009). Tested solutions for eliminating Canada's registered nurse

shortage. Ottawa, Canada: Canadian Nurses Association. Downloaded 4 April 2018 from

https://www.cna-aiic.ca/en/news-room/news-releases/2009/eliminating-canadas-rn-

shortage

Centers for Medicare & Medicaid Services (2018). Therapy Services. Downloaded 5 July 2018

from *https://www.cms.gov/Medicare/Billing/TherapyServices/index.html*

Chamove, A. S., & Anderson, J. R. (1989). Examining environmental enrichment. Park Ridge,

NJ: Noyes Publications.

Chang, T. R., Forthman, D. L., & Maple, T. L. (1999). Comparison of confined mandrill

(Mandrillus sphinx) behavior in traditional and "ecologically representative"

exhibits. *Zoo Biology, 18*(3), 163-176.

Chatchawan, U., Eungpinichpong, W., Plandee, P., & Yamauchi, J. (2015). Effects of thai foot

massage on balance performance in diabetic patients with peripheral neuropathy: a

randomized parallel-controlled trial. *Medical Science Monitor Basic Research, 21*, 68.

Cohen, S. (2004). Social relationships and health. *American Psychologist, 59,* 676–684.

Cohen, S., Doyle, W. J., Skoner, D. P., Rabin, B. S., & Gwaltney, J. M., Jr. (1997). Social ties

and susceptibility to the common cold. *Journal of the American Medical Association,

277,* 1940–1944.

Couck, M. D., Marechal, R., Moorthamers, S., Laethem, J. L., & Gidron, Y. (2016). Vagal nerve

activity predicts overall survival in metastatic pancreatic cancer, mediated by

inflammation. *Cancer Epidemiology, 40,* 47-51.

Dane, E., & Brummel, B. J. (2014). Examining workplace mindfulness and its relations to job performance and turnover intention. *Human Relations, 67*(1), 105-128.

DeVore, S., Winchell, B., & Rowe, J. M. (2016). Intergenerational programming for young children and older adults: An overview of needs, approaches, and outcomes in the United States. *Childhood Education, 92*(3), 216-225.

Diego, M. A., Field, T., Sanders, C., & Hernandez-Reif, M. (2004). Massage therapy of moderate and light pressure and vibrator effects on EEG and heart rate. *International Journal of Neuroscience, 114*(1), 31-44.

Dixon, K. E., Keefe, F. J., Scipio, C. D., Perri, L. M., & Abernethy, A. P. (2007). Psychological interventions for arthritis pain management in adults: a meta-analysis. *Health Psychology, 26*(3), 241.

Duggan, K., & Julliard, K. (2018). Implementation of a mindfulness moment initiative for healthcare professionals: Perceptions of facilitators. *Explore: The Journal of Science and Healing, 14*(1), 44-58.

Dunbar, R. I., & Shultz, S. (2007). Evolution in the social brain. Science, 317, 1344–1347.

Dupuy, O., Douzi, W., Theurot, D., Bosquet, L., & Dugué, B. (2018). An evidence-based approach for choosing post-exercise recovery techniques to reduce markers of muscle damage, soreness, fatigue and inflammation: a systematic review with meta-analysis. *Frontiers in Physiology, 9*, 403.

Epstein, A. S., & Boisvert, C. (2006). Let's do something together: Identifying the effective

    components of intergenerational programs. *Journal of Intergenerational Relationships,*

    *4(*3), 87-109.

Fabes, R. A., Eisenberg, N., & Eisenbud, L. (1993). Behavioral and physiological correlates of

    children's reactions to others in distress. Developmental Psychology, 29, 655–663.

Falcone, G., & Jerram, M. (2018). Brain activity in mindfulness depends on experience: a meta-

    analysis of fMRI studies. *Mindfulness*, 1-11.

Fan, Y., Tang, Y. Y., & Posner, M. I. (2014). Cortisol level modulated by integrative meditation

    in a dose-dependent fashion. *Stress and Health, 30*(1), 65-70.

Femia, E., Zarit, S., Blair, C., Jarrott, S., & Bruno, K. (2008). Intergenerational preschool

    experiences and the young child: Potential benefits to development. *Early Childhood*

    Research Quarterly, 23(2), 272-287.

Femia, E., Zarit, S., Blair, C., Jarrott, S., & Bruno, K. (2008). Intergenerational preschool

    experiences and the young child: Potential benefits to development. *Early Childhood*

    Research Quarterly, 23(2), 272-287.

Field, T. (2011). Yoga clinical research review. *Complementary Therapies in Clinical*

    Practice, 17(1), 1-8.

Field, T., Diego, M., Delgado, J., & Medina, L. (2013). Tai chi/yoga reduces prenatal depression,

    anxiety and sleep disturbances. *Complementary Therapies in Clinical Practice, 19*(1), 6-

    10.

Flora, P. & Faulkner, G. (2007). Physical activity: An innovative context for intergenerational programming. *Journal of Intergenerational Relationships, 4*(4), 63-74.

Fox, K. C., Dixon, M. L., Nijeboer, S., Girn, M., Floman, J. L., Lifshitz, M., ... & Christoff, K. (2016). Functional neuroanatomy of meditation: A review and meta-analysis of 78 functional neuroimaging investigations. *Neuroscience & Biobehavioral Reviews, 65*, 208-228.

Fox, K.C., Nijeboer, S., Dixon, M., Floman, J.L., Ellamil, B., Rumak, R., ... & Christoff, K. (2014). Is meditation associated with altered brain structure? A systematic review and meta-analysis of morphometric neuroimaging in meditation practitioners. *Neuroscience and Biobehavioral Reviews, 43*, 48-73.

Francis, R. (2013). *Report of the Mid Staffordshire NHS Foundation Trust Public Inquiry.* London: The Stationery Office.

Fredin, K., & Lorås, H. (2017). Manual therapy, exercise therapy or combined treatment in the management of adult neck pain–A systematic review and meta-analysis. *Musculoskeletal Science and Practice, 31*, 62-71.

George Mason University (2015). Medicare's role in determining prices throughout the health care system. *Mercatus Center.* Downloaded 5 July 2018 from https://www.mercatus.org/publication/medicare-role-determining-prices-throughout-health-care-system

Gigliotti, C., Morris, M., Smock, S., Jarrott, S., & Graham, B. (2005). An intergenerational summer program involving persons with dementia and preschool children. *Educational Gerontology, 31*(6), 425-441.

Gilbert, C., & Ricketts, K. (2008). Children's attitudes towards older adults and aging: A synthesis of research. *Educational Gerontology, 34,* 370-386.

Glomb, T.M., Duffy, M. K., Bono, J. E., & Yang, T. (2011). Mindfulness at work. *Research on Personnel Human Resources Management, 30,* 115.

Good, D. J., Lyddy, C. J., Glomb, T. M., Bono, J. E., Brown, K. W., Duffy, M. K., ... & Lazar, S. W. (2016). Contemplating mindfulness at work: An integrative review. *Journal of Management, 42*(1), 114-142.

Greeson, J., & Brantley, J. (2009). Mindfulness and anxiety disorders: Developing a wise relationship with the inner experience of fear. In F. Didonna (Ed.), Clinical handbook of mindfulness (pp. 171–188). New York, NY: Springer.

Guleria, R., Arora, S., Mohan, A., Kumar, G., & Kumar, A. (2015). Yoga is as effective as standard pulmonary rehabilitation in improving dyspnea, inflammatory markers, and quality of life in patients with COPD. *Chest, 148*(4), 907A.

Hall, A., Copsey, B., Richmond, H., Thompson, J., Ferreira, M., Latimer, J., & Maher, C. G. (2017). Effectiveness of tai chi for chronic musculoskeletal pain conditions: updated systematic review and meta-analysis. *Physical Therapy, 97*(2), 227-238.

Harris, A. R., Jennings, P. A., Katz, D. A., Abenavoli, R. M., & Greenberg, M. T. (2016).

Promoting stress management and wellbeing in educators: Feasibility and efficacy of a

school-based yoga and mindfulness intervention. *Mindfulness, 7*(1), 143-154.

Harvard Medical School. (2008). *Now and Zen.* Longwood Seminar, 2008. Downloaded on 12

March 2018 from https://youtu.be/9MYvhJsmggA

Hayes, C. (2003). An observational study in developing an intergenerational shared site program:

Challenges and insights. *Journal of Intergenerational Relationships, 1*(1), 113-132.

Hayhurst, C. (2015). *Measuring by value, not volume.* PT in Motion, APTA. Downloaded 7 July

2018 from http://www.apta.org/PTinMotion/2015/7/Feature/MeasuringByValue/

Hernandez-Reif, M., Field, T., Ironson, G., Beutler, J., Vera, Y., Hurley, J., ... & Hernandez-

Reif, M. (2005). Natural killer cells and lymphocytes increase in women with breast

cancer following massage therapy. *International Journal of Neuroscience, 115*(4), 495-

510.

Hernandez-Reif, M., Ironson, G., Field, T., Hurley, J., Katz, G., Diego, M., ... & Burman, I.

(2004). Breast cancer patients have improved immune and neuroendocrine functions

following massage therapy. *Journal of Psychosomatic Research, 57*(1), 45-52.

Heyman, J. C., Gutheil, I. A., & White-Ryan, L. (2011). Preschool children's attitudes toward

older adults: Comparison of intergenerational and traditional day care. *Journal of

Intergenerational Relationships, 9*(4), 435- 444.

Hilton, L., Hempel, S., Ewing, B. A., Apaydin, E., Xenakis, L., Newberry, S., ... & Maglione, M.
A. (2016). Mindfulness meditation for chronic pain: systematic review and meta-
analysis. *Annals of Behavioral Medicine, 51*(2), 199-213.

Holmes, C. (2009). An intergenerational program with benefits. *Early Childhood Education
Journal, 37,* 113-119.

Holmes, C. (2009). An intergenerational program with benefits. *Early Childhood Education
Journal, 37,* 113-119.

Holt-Lunstad, J., Smith, T. B., & Layton, J. B. (2010). Social relationships and mortality risk: A
meta-analytic review. *PLoS Medicine, 7,* e1000316.

Holt-Lunstad, J., Smith, T. B., & Layton, J. B. (2010). Social relationships and mortality risk: A
meta-analytic review. *PLoS Medicine, 7,* e1000316.

Hölzel, B. K., Carmody, J., Vangel, M., Congleton, C., Yerramsetti, S. M., Gard, T., & Lazar, S.
W. (2011). Mindfulness practice leads to increases in regional brain gray matter
density. *Psychiatry Research: Neuroimaging, 191*(1), 36-43.

Horney, K. (1950). *Neurosis and human growth.* New York, NY: W.W. Norton & Company.

Hossain, M. S., Rahman, M. A., & Muhammad, G. (2017). Towards energy-aware cloud-
oriented cyber-physical therapy system. *Future Generation Computer Systems.*

Hülsheger, U. R., Alberts, H. J., Feinholdt, A., & Lang, J. W. (2013). Benefits of mindfulness at
work: the role of mindfulness in emotion regulation, emotional exhaustion, and job
satisfaction. *Journal of Applied Psychology, 98*(2), 310.

Institute of Medicine (2004). *Improving medical education: Enhancing the behavioral and social science content of medical school curricula.* Washington, DC: National Academies Press.

Jang, J. H., Jung, W. H., Kang, D. H., Byun, M. S., Kwon, S. J., Choi, C. H., & Kwon, J. S. (2011). Increased default mode network connectivity associated with meditation. *Neuroscience Letters, 487*(3), 358-362.

Jarrott, S., & Bruno, K. (2007). Shared site intergenerational programs: A case study. *Journal of Applied Gerontology, 26*(3), 239-257.

Jarrott, S., Smith, C., & Weintraub, A. (2008). Development of a standardized tool for intergenerational programming: The intergenerational observation scale. *Journal of Intergenerational Relationships, 6*(4), 433-447.

Job openings and labor turnover (2018). *Bureau of Labor and Statistics; U.S. Department of Labor.* Downloaded 9 July 2018 form https://www.bls.gov/news.release/pdf/jolts.pdf

Jongman-Sereno, K. (2017). Personality and self-knowledge. Cambridge, MA: Harvard University, Psyc E-1707.

Jongman-Sereno, K. (2017). Personality and self-knowledge. Cambridge, MA: Harvard University, Psyc E-1707.

Jongman-Sereno, K. (2017). Personality and self-knowledge. *Cambridge, MA: Harvard University, Psychology,* E-1707.

Kabat-Zinn, J. (2013). *What is mindfulness?.* [video] (5:17). Downloaded 3 March 2018 from https://www.youtube.com/watch?v=HmEo6RI4Wvs

Kalyani, B., Venkatasubramanian, G., Arasappa, R., Rao, N., Kalmady, S., Behere, R., ... &
Gangadhar, B. (2011). Neuro-hemodynamic correlates of 'OM' chanting: A pilot
functional magnetic resonance imaging study. *International Journal of Yoga, 4*(1), 3-6.

Kayser, C., & Shams, L. (2015). Multisensory causal inference in the brain. *PLoS biology, 13*(2),
e1002075.

Kemp, A. H., Quintana, D. S., Kuhnert, R., Griffiths, K., Hickie, I. B., & Guastella, A. J. (2012).
Oxytocin increases heart rate variability in humans at rest: Implications for social
approach-related motivation and capacity for social engagement. PLoS ONE, 7, e44014.
Retrieved from http://www .plosone.org/article/info:doi/10.1371/journal.pone.0044014

Kemper, K.J., Mo, X., & Khayat, R. (2015). Are mindfulness and self-compassion associated
with sleep and resilience in health professionals? Journal of Alternative and
Complementary Medicine, 21(8), 496–503.

Kim, T. Y., Bateman, T. S., Gilbreath, B. & Andersson, L. M. (2009). Top management
credibility and employee cynicism: a comprehensive model. *Human Relations, 62,* 1435–
1458.

King, A., Angstadt, M., Sripada, C., & Liberzon, I. (2017). Increased default mode network
(DMN) connectivity with attention networks with a mindfulness-based intervention for
PTSD: seed and whole brain connectomics analyses. *Biological Psychiatry, 81*(10), S43-
S44.

Kok, B. E., Coffey, K. A., Cohn, M. A., Catalino, L. I., Vacharkulksemsuk, T., Algoe, S. B., ...
& Fredrickson, B. L. (2013). How positive emotions build physical health perceived

positive social connections account for the upward spiral between positive emotions and vagal tone. *Psychological Science, 24*(7), 1123-1132.

Lamprecht, R., & LeDoux, J. (2004). Structural plasticity and memory. *Nature Reviews Neuroscience, 5*(1), 45.

Langer, E.J. (2012). *Counterclockwise: the power of possibility.* [video] (25:23). Downloaded on 18 March 2018 from *https://www.youtube.com/watch?v=fZffBAefwUM.*

Leary, M. R., Tate, E. B., Adams, C. E., Allen, A. B., & Hancock, J. (2007). Self-compassion and reactions to unpleasant events: The implications of treating oneself kindly. Journal of Personality and Social Psychology, 92, 887–904.

Leary, M. R., Tate, E. B., Adams, C. E., Batts Allen, A., & Hancock, J. (2007). Self-compassion and reactions to unpleasant self-relevant events: the implications of treating oneself kindly. *Journal of personality and social psychology, 92*(5), 887.

Lee, A. C., Harvey, W. F., Wong, J. B., Price, L. L., Han, X., Chung, M., ... & Wang, C. (2017). Effects of tai chi versus physical therapy on mindfulness in knee osteoarthritis. *Mindfulness, 8*(5), 1195-1205.

Leonardi, R., Buchanan-Smith, H. M., Dufour, V., MacDonald, C., & Whiten, A. (2010). Living together: Behaviour and welfare in single and mixed species groups of capuchin (Cebus apella) and squirrel monkeys (Saimiri sciureus). American Journal of Primatology, 72, 33–47.

Leroy, H., Anseel, F., Dimitrova, N. G., & Sels, L. (2013). Mindfulness, authentic functioning, and work engagement: A growth modeling approach. *Journal of Vocational Behavior, 82*(3), 238-247.

Lindahl, J. R., Fisher, N. E., Cooper, D. J., Rosen, R. K., & Britton, W. B. (2017). The varieties of contemplative experience: A mixed-methods study of meditation-related challenges in western Buddhists. *PloS One, 12*(5).

Lucas, A. R., Klepin, H. D., Porges, S. W., & Rejeski, W. J. (2016). Mindfulness-based movement: a polyvagal perspective. *Integrative Cancer Therapies*, 1534735416682087.

Luksyte, E., Spitzmeuller, C., & Maynard, D.C. (2011). Why do overqualified incumbents deviate? Examining multiple mediators. *Journal of Occupational Health Psychology, 16,* 279–296.

Lynott, P., & Merola, P. (2007). Improving the attitudes of 4th graders toward older people through a multidimensional intergenerational program. *Educational Gerontology, 33*(1), 63-74.

MacLean, R. (2014). The Vale of Leven Hospital Inquiry. Retrieved 5 August 2016 from *www.valeoflevenhospitalinquiry.org.*

Magnon ,C., Hall, S. J., & Lin, J. (2013). Autonomic nerve development contributes to prostate cancer progression. *Science, 341*:1236361.

Mak, L. E., Minuzzi, L., MacQueen, G., Hall, G., Kennedy, S. H., & Milev, R. (2017). The default mode network in healthy individuals: a systematic review and meta-analysis. *Brain Connectivity, 7*(1), 25-33.

Mantler, J., Godin, J., Cameron, S. J., & Horsburgh, M. E. (2015). Cynicism in hospital staff

    nurses: The effect of intention to leave and job change over time. *Journal of Nursing*

    Management, 23(5), 577-587.

Maratos, F. A., Duarte, J., Barnes, C., McEwan, K., Sheffield, D., & Gilbert, P. (2017). The

    physiological and emotional effects of touch: Assessing a hand-massage intervention

    with high self-critics. *Psychiatry Research, 250*, 221-227.

Marcel, D., Kozasa, E., Afonso, R., Galduroz, J., Leite, J. (2015). Yoga and compassion

    meditation program improve quality of life and self-compassion in family caregivers of

    Alzheimer's disease patients: A randomized controlled trial. Geriatrics Gerontology, Int;

    17: 85–91.

Martire, L. M., & Franks, M. M. (2014). The role of social networks in adult health: Introduction

    to the special issue. *Health Psychology, 33*(6), 501.

Maslach, C., & Leiter, M. P. (2016). Understanding the burnout experience: recent research and

    its implications for psychiatry. *World Psychiatry, 15*(2), 103-111.

McConville, J., McAleer, R., & Hahne, A. (2017). Mindfulness training for health profession

    students—the effect of mindfulness training on psychological well-being, learning and

    clinical performance of health professional students: a systematic review of randomized

    and non-randomized controlled trials. *Explore: The Journal of Science and*

    Healing, 13(1), 26-45.

Middlecamp, M., & Gross, D. (2002). Intergenerational daycare and preschoolers' attitudes

    about aging. *Educational Gerontology, 28*(4), 271-288.

Mileski, M., Topinka, J. B., Lee, K., Brooks, M., McNeil, C., & Jackson, J. (2017). An

investigation of quality improvement initiatives in decreasing the rate of avoidable 30-

day, skilled nursing facility-to-hospital readmissions: a systematic review. *Clinical

interventions in aging, 12,* 213.

Moodie, E. M., & Chamove, A. S. (1990). Brief threatening events beneficial for captive

tamarins? Zoo Biology, 9, 69 275–286.

Neff, K. D. (2003). The development and validation of a scale to measure self-compassion. Self

and Identity, 2, 223–250.

Neff, K. D., Kirkpatrick, K., & Rude, S. S. (2007). Self-compassion and its link to adaptive

psychological functioning. Journal of Research in Personality, 41, 139–154.

Nelson, N. L. (2015). Massage therapy: understanding the mechanisms of action on blood

pressure. A scoping review. *Journal of the American Society of Hypertension, 9*(10), 785-

793.

Ng, L., Chiang, L. K., Tang, R., Siu, C., Fung, L., Lee, A., & Tam, W. (2014). Effectiveness of

incorporating Tai Chi in a pulmonary rehabilitation program for Chronic Obstructive

Pulmonary Disease (COPD) in primary care—A pilot randomized controlled

trial. *European Journal of Integrative Medicine, 6*(3), 248-258.

Nielsen, M., Keefe, F. J., Bennell, K., & Jull, G. A. (2014). PT–delivered cognitive-behavioral

therapy: a qualitative study of PTs' perceptions and experiences. *Physical therapy, 94*(2),

197-209.

Nielsen, M., Keefe, F. J., Bennell, K., & Jull, G. A. (2014). PT–delivered cognitive-behavioral therapy: a qualitative study of PTs' perceptions and experiences. *Physical therapy*, *94*(2), 197-209.

Noseworthy, J. (2017). *10 prominent health system CEOs: Physician burnout is a public health crisis — here are 11 things we commit to do about it.* Becker's Hospital Review. Downloaded 7 July 2018 from https://www.beckershospitalreview.com/hospital-physician-relationships/ceos-of-mayo-cleveland-clinic-partners-and-other-health-systems-pen-call-to-action-on-physician-burnout.html

Offord, N., Wyrko, Z., Downes, T., Hopper, A., Harriman, P., & Gordon, A. L. (2016). Frailsafe: from conception to national breakthrough collaborative. *Acute medicine*, *15*(3), 134-139.

Olson, K., Kemper, K.J., & Mahan, J.D. (2015). What factors promote resilience and protect against burnout in first-year pediatric and medicine-pediatric residents? Journal of Evidence-Based Complementary & Alternative Medicine, 20(3), 192–198.

Pasquaretta, C., Levé, M., Claidiere, N., van de Waal, E., Whiten, A., …Sueur, C. (2014). Social networks in primates: Smart and tolerant species have more efficient networks. Scientific Reports, 4, 7600.

Patsiopoulos, A.T., & Buchanan, M.J. (2011). The practice of self-compassion in counseling: A narrative inquiry. Professional Psychology: Research and Practice, 42, 301–307.

Physical Therapy Workforce Project: Physical Therapy Vacancy and Turnover Rates in Skilled Nursing Facilities. Alexandria, VA: *American Physical Therapy Association*; 2008.

Porges, S. W. (2007). The polyvagal perspective. Biological Psychology, 74, 116–143.

Putnam, D. E., Finney, J. W., Barkley, P. L., & Bonner, M. J. (1994). Enhancing commitment improves adherence to a medical regimen. Journal of Consulting and Clinical Psychology, 62, 191–194.

Reuter, M., Tisdall, M. D., Qureshi, A., Buckner, R. L., van der Kouwe, A. J., & Fischl, B. (2015). Head motion during MRI acquisition reduces gray matter volume and thickness estimates. *NeuroImage, 107,* 107–115.

Reyna, C., Goodwin, E. J., & Ferrari, J. R. (2007). Older adult stereotypes among care providers in residential care facilities: Examining the relationship between con- tact, education, and ageism. *Journal of Gerontological Nursing, 33*(2), 50-55.

Riley, K. E., & Park, C. L. (2015). How does yoga reduce stress? A systematic review of mechanisms of change and guide to future inquiry. *Health Psychology Review, 9*(3), 379-396.

Rook, K. S., August, K. J., & Sorkin, D. H. (2011). Social network functions and health. In R. Contrada & A. Baum (Eds.), *Handbook of stress science: Biology, psychology, and health* (pp. 123–135). New York, NY: Springer.

Rose Ru-Whui, L., Sung, Y., & Chang, K. (2013). Game-induced learning effect: A cognitive neuroscience perspective. In *Proceedings of the 2013 International Conference on Information, Business and Education Technology (ICIBET 2013)*. Atlantis Press.

Rose, P. E., & Croft, D. P. (2015). The potential of Social Network Analysis as a tool for the management of zoo animals. *Animal Welfare, 24*(2), 123-138.

Rubin, S. (2016). Palette: An intergenerational art program to improve health care delivery and health outcomes of older adults. *Age in Action, 31*(1), 1.

Salari, S. (2002). Intergenerational partnerships in adult day centers: Importance of age-appropriate environments and behaviors. *The Gerontologist, 42*(3), 321.

Schilling, R. (2017). Relaxation reduces inflammation. Downloaded on 10 July 2018 from https://www.askdrray.com/relaxation-reduces-inflammation/

Scoglio, A., Rudat, D., Garvert, D., Jamolowski, M., Jackson, C., Herman, J. (2015). Self-compassiona and responses to trauma: the role of emotion regulation. Journal of Interpersonal Violence, 1-21.

Senyuva, E., Kaya, H., Isik, B., & Bodur, G. (2014). Relationship between self-compassion and emotional intelligence in nursing students. International Journal of Nursing Practice, 20, 588–596.

Shapiro, D. (1992). Adverse effects of meditation: a preliminary investigation of long-term meditators. *International Journal of Psychosomatics, 39*, 62-67.

Shapiro, S. L., & Schwartz, G. E. R. (1999). Intentional systematic mindfulness: An integrative model for self-regulation and health. Advances in Mind-Body Medicine, 15, 128–134.

Shin, L. M., & Liberzon, I. (2010). The Neurocircuitry of Fear, Stress, and Anxiety Disorders. *Neuropsychopharmacology, 35*(1), 169–191.

Short-DeGraff, M., & Diamond, K. (1996). Intergenerational program effects on social responses of elderly adult day care members. *Educational Gerontology, 22*(5), 467.

Singer, D. G., Golinkoff, R. M., & Hirsh-Pasek, K. (Eds.). (2006). *Play= Learning: How play motivates and enhances children's cognitive and social-emotional growth.* Oxford, UK: Oxford University Press.

Sodaro, V. (1999). Housing and exhibition of mixed species of Neotropical primates. Brookfield, IL: Chicago Zoological Society.

Song, N., Liu, J., Proctor, M., & Yu, J. (2015). Right and left vagus nerves regulate breathing by multiplicative interaction. *Respiratory Physiology & Neurobiology, 219*, 25-29.

Steptoe, A., Shankar, A., Demakakos, P., & Wardle, J. (2013). Social isolation, loneliness, and all-cause mortality in older men and women. *Proceedings of the National Academy of Sciences, 110*(15), 5797-5801.

Sullivan, M. B., Erb, M., Schmalzl, L., Moonaz, S., Noggle Taylor, J., Porges, S. W., & Porges, S. W. (2018). Yoga therapy and polyvagal theory: the convergence of traditional wisdom and contemporary neuroscience for self-regulation and resilience. *Frontiers in Human Neuroscience, 12*, 67.

Taylor, L. M., Kerse, N., Frakking, T., & Maddison, R. (2018). Active video games for improving physical performance measures in older people: a meta-analysis. *Journal of Geriatric Physical Therapy (2001), 41*(2), 108.

Tejero-Fernández, V., Membrilla-Mesa, M., Galiano-Castillo, N., & Arroyo-Morales, M. (2015). Immunological effects of massage after exercise: A systematic review. *Physical Therapy in Sport, 16*(2), 187-192.

Thayer, J. F., & Sternberg, E. (2006). Beyond heart rate variability: Vagal regulation of allostatic systems. *Annals of the New York Academy of Sciences, 1088*, 361-372.

The Commission on Affordable Housing and Health Facility Needs for Seniors in the 21st Century (2002). Intergenerational learning and care centers. *Generations United.* Downloaded on 6 July 2018 from https://govinfo.library.unt.edu/seniorscommission/pages/final_report/generationsUnited.html

Thompson, D. (2017). *Be 'mindful' of the hype; Scientists call for rigorous research to back up mindfulness marketing claims.* Consumer Health News. Downloaded 4 April 2018 from https://consumer.healthday.com/alternative-medicine-information-3/meditation-news-467/be-mindful-of-the-hype-727395.html

Throop, C. J. (2010). *Suffering and sentiment: Exploring the vicissitudes of experience and pain in Yap.* University of California Press.

Tsang, H. W., Chan, E. P., & Cheung, W. M. (2008). Effects of mindful and non-mindful exercises on people with depression: a systematic review. *British Journal of Clinical Psychology, 47*(3), 303-322.

University of New Mexico (2016). *The cost of losing nurses.* Downloaded 4 April 2018 from https://rnbsnonline.unm.edu/articles/high-cost-of-nurse-turnover.aspx

Van Dam, N. T., van Vugt, M. K., Vago, D. R., Schmalzl, L., Saron, C. D., Olendzki, A., ... & Fox, K. C. (2018). Mind the hype: A critical evaluation and prescriptive agenda for research on mindfulness and meditation. *Perspectives on Psychological Science, 13*(1), 36-61.

Van Muijden, J., Band, G.P. & Hommel, B. (2012). Online games training aging brains: Limited transfer to cognitive control functions. *Frontiers in Human Neuroscience, 6,* 221.

Vanderkooi, L. (1997). Buddhist teachers' experience with extreme mental states in western meditators. *Journal of Transpersonal Psychology, 29,* 31-46.

Veasey, J., & Hammer, G. (2010). Managing captive mammals in mixed species communities. In D. G. Kleiman, K. V. Thompson, & C. Kirk Baer (Eds.), Wild mammals in captivity: Principles and techniques (pp. 151–161). Chicago, IL: University of Chicago Press.

Volkman, J. (2018). Neuroscience of learning: an introduction to mind, brain, health, and education. *Cambridge, MA: Harvard University,* Psychology, E-1609.

Wanous, J. P., Reichers, A. E., & Austin, J. T. (2000). Cynicism about organizational change: measurement, antecedents, and correlates. *Group and Organization Management, 25,* 132– 153.

Wei, G. X., Li, Y. F., Yue, X. L., Ma, X., Chang, Y. K., Yi, L. Y., ... & Zuo, X. N. (2016). Tai Chi Chuan modulates heart rate variability during abdominal breathing in elderly adults. *PsyCh journal, 5*(1), 69-77.

Willis, L. (2015). Raising the bar: The shape of caring review. London: Health Education England.

Wong, R., Odom, C. J., & Barr, J. O. (2014). Building the physical therapy workforce for an aging America. *Journal of Physical Therapy Education, 28*(2), 12-21.

Yoo, Y. G., Lee, D. J., Lee, I. S., Shin, N., Park, J. Y., Yoon, M. R., & Yu, B. (2016). The effects of mind subtraction meditation on depression, social anxiety, aggression, and salivary cortisol levels of elementary school children in South Korea. *Journal of pediatric nursing, 31*(3), e185-e197.

Young, K. S., van der Velden, A. M., Craske, M. G., Pallesen, K. J., Fjorback, L., Roepstorff, A., & Parsons, C. E. (2017). The impact of mindfulness-based interventions on brain activity: a systematic review of functional magnetic resonance imaging studies. *Neuroscience & Biobehavioral Reviews, 84*, 424-433.

Yuan, S. L. K., Matsutani, L. A., & Marques, A. P. (2015). Effectiveness of different styles of massage therapy in fibromyalgia: a systematic review and meta-analysis. *Manual Therapy, 20*(2), 257-264.

Zeidan, F., Emerson, N. M., Farris, S. R., Ray, J. N., Jung, Y., McHaffie, J. G., & Coghill, R. C. (2015). Mindfulness meditation-based pain relief employs different neural mechanisms than placebo and sham mindfulness meditation-induced analgesia. *Journal of Neuroscience, 35*(46), 15307-15325.

Zeng, Y., Luo, T., Xie, H., Huang, M., & Cheng, A. S. (2014). Health benefits of qigong or tai chi for cancer patients: a systematic review and meta-analyses. *Complementary therapies in medicine, 22*(1), 173-186.

Zimmerman, K. (2016). Immune system: disease, disorder and dysfunction. *Live Science.* Downloaded on 9 March 2018 from https://www.livescience.com/26579-immune-system.html

Zou, L., Wang, H., Xiao, Z., Fang, Q., Zhang, M., Li, T., ... & Liu, Y. (2017). Tai chi for health

benefits in patients with multiple sclerosis: A systematic review. *PloS one, 12*(2),

e0170212.